DAVID BOWEN is Emeritus Professor of Forensic Medicine at the University of London. Born in Pontycymmer, Wales in 1924, he studied medicine at Cardiff, Cambridge and Middlesex Hospital, London. Training in House Officer posts led to training in clinical pathology and histopathology at the Royal Marsden Hospital. A chance vacancy at St George's Hospital opened the way to join the late Donald Teare in 1956. Ten years later he moved to Charing Cross Hospital Medical School, starting the Department of Forensic Medicine, becoming Reader and then, in 1977, Professor.

He has been involved in some 500 murder and suspicious death investigations as a Home Office Coroner and Medical School Pathologist. During the course of work he has travelled and lectured in Europe, India, Sri Lanka, Jordan, Egypt, the United States and Canada, and has been appointed Examiner of Forensic Medicine at the University of Saudi Arabia and at the University of Colombo, Sri Lanka.

BODY
of
EVIDENCE

DAVID BOWEN

ROBINSON
London

Constable & Robinson Ltd
3 The Lanchesters
162 Fulham Palace Road
London W6 9ER
www.constablerobinson.com

First published in the UK by Constable,
an imprint of Constable & Robinson Ltd 2003

This paperback edition published by Robinson,
an imprint of Constable & Robinson Ltd 2003

A copy of the British Library Cataloguing in
Publication Data is available from the British Library

ISBN 1-84119-739-4 (pbk)
ISBN 1-84119-628-2 (hbk)

Printed and bound in the EU

10 9 8 7 6 5 4 3 2 1

Contents

Illustrations

Site of discovery of body.
Metropolitan Police

Peter Thomas's body in a shallow grave.
Curator, Thames Valley Police Museum

The Chamber of Shipping building in the City of London after an IRA bomb.
Press Association

Aircraft crash at Heathrow.
London Fire Brigade Library

Scaffolding at Blackfriars Bridge where Calvi's body was found.
City of London Police

Passport found in Calvi's clothing.
City of London Police

Unsolved murder, Amersham, Buckinghamshire.
Curator, Thames Valley Police Museum

Moundis, the man accused of Ann Chapman's murder.
Edward Chapman

Ann Chapman's body in a sheep fold near Athens.
Edward Chapman.

Preface

The role of the forensic pathologist is well known, mainly through television plays, documentaries and reconstructions of *causes célèbres*. Forensic pathology remains a small branch of medicine but is an exciting and rigorous discipline, requiring an all-round knowledge of pathology and an ability to present medical evidence in courts of law. Nowadays there are links with anthropology, archaeology, odontology and radiology, but medical detection still plays a vital part in solving a crime. The pathologist's ability to recognize and interpret forensic clues remains paramount, but is part of a team effort; the 'big chief' image beloved of yore no longer pertains.

Before attempting to obtain a post in forensic pathology it is necessary to obtain training and experience in ordinary pathology. Training is straightforward, in the sense that junior posts, preferably in teaching hospitals, provide an excellent framework basis for the acquisition of an understanding of all forms of disease processes. (It is sometimes forgotten that ninety per cent of a forensic pathologist's work is concerned with the evaluation and diagnosis of natural death and, in particular, non-suspicious death; investigations into unnatural death are only a small part of it all.) Not so straightforward, after one has trained for several years in all branches of pathology, is the matter of finding a post. Nowadays there are very few satisfactory career-structure posts available.

Despite considerable interest in forensic matters through detective novels and television series, media interest in pathologists has waned over the years; certainly today we see no headlines like the traditional 'SPILSBURY CALLED IN'. Years ago I went with Donald Teare to a terraced house in Acton and, emerging after his survey of the scene inside – it wasn't an out-of-the-ordinary murder – he faced a number of reporters and camera flashes . . . and this was late in the afternoon on a wintry day! Modern newspaper and court reports of murder investigations do not so often include the pathologist's name as in the past (although local reporters still attend almost all inquests in the hope of generating good copy for the following day's edition).

On a lighter note, during the Dennis Nilsen trial, a psychiatrist was called to give evidence on Nilsen's state of mind. I myself did not testify in person as my testimony had been presented and accepted as documentary evidence. During the course of the trial an account appeared in the *Evening Standard* of the enormous task that had had to be undertaken in the quest for identification of victims, and immediately above it was a photograph purporting to be of the forensic pathologist, Professor Bowen – me. In fact, it was of the psychiatrist, a Dr Bowden – far better looking than myself.

Careers in medicine are often fashioned by chance. In my case, my career was the result of a phone call and an interview, leading to an opportunity to 'carry the bag' for a well known London forensic pathologist. By this time I had spent ten years in clinical medicine and hospital pathology, so my new appointment was, on paper, a junior post, but the challenge to leave a cloistered life for an entrepreneurial one was considerable: it was exchanging a white coat and microscope for a mortuary gown and post-mortem table.

Ah, yes, the post-mortem table. Occasionally friends query the ambience of autopsy examinations and I remind them of the surgeon's day in a hot theatre, opening body cavities, dissecting and excising tissues to eradicate disease. The forensic pathologist may be considered to have something of a surgeon's approach to his or her work – dissecting tissues and noting minimal but vital changes in organs – but without the urgency: after all, your patient's not going to die on you. Both surgeon and forensic pathologist, if they are in demand, lead very active lives with limited time for other activities. Forensic pathologists spend time outside the mortuary meeting colleagues over autopsies, attending conferences and discussing findings with coroners, lawyers and senior detectives. There are few routine cases; witness, as just one very common example, the varying presentation of heart attacks, which can be unheralded and misdiagnosed until the autopsy. In murder and suspicious deaths one has to be quite sure of one's findings, as in many cases the true nature of a person's death may be concealed amid information supplied by witnesses.

During the course of my work I have seen many changes, the most fundamental being the use of DNA which has proved, time and again, vital in solving murders and other crimes. As a result, the pathologist has to be even more careful in his examination at the scene of a suspected crime in preserving and collecting evidence for forensic scientists.

The three senior pathologists of my time – Camps, Simpson and Teare – had established departments which are no longer. Whilst forensic medicine has flourished through the Association of Police Surgeons, forensic pathology, particularly in London, has suffered from lack of academic and research facilities. Nowadays in the capital city small groups of experienced forensic pathologists operate in 'medical chambers' available to the police and coroners to investigate murder and suspicious death but forensic pathology awaits a career structure, particularly in

London. Outside London there are departments in Cardiff, Sheffield and Scotland under university aegis. Hope for a new structure of the subject may be in the Home Office Enquiry into Death Certification which includes the role of the pathologist.

I hope that this book about my career and my most interesting cases will succeed in its aim of introducing you to the world of the forensic pathologist – at least, the world of this particular forensic pathologist.

David Bowen

Chapter One

A Case to Remember

It ain't over until the fat lady sings – an apt enough saying in the case of the Railway Murders, as that *cause célèbre* became known. One man, John Duffy, had been charged and convicted of two murders in 1988, two years after the crimes had taken place. It was not until September 2000 that a second man, Duffy's close friend David Mulcahy, stood trial on the same charges.

So I was once more at the Central Criminal Court to give my evidence on the last of the three murders. As I left the court and walked down the broad stairway at the Old Bailey I reflected on some forty years spent as a forensic pathologist investigating suspicious deaths and murders, on behalf of both the coroner and the CID.

I became involved in the investigation of the Railway Murders one warm July day in 1986, when I was called by the coroner's officer for the district, to view and examine a body found by men working on a railway embankment between Potters Bar and Brookmans Park in Hertfordshire, north of London. The decomposed body was in undergrowth adjacent to the main line between London and the north of England, at the side of a pathway between the embankment and an area of scrubland.

My preliminary examination showed a body just visible in the long grass, surrounded by weeds. It was clear that the body had lain in that area for some time. I arranged to return after a modicum of scrub had been cleared.

Some distance away, a group of Hertfordshire Police officers craned over the parapet of the bridge across the railway line at Brookmans Park station. Their presence and interest were based on the extensive investigation that had been carried out by both the Metropolitan and the Hertfordshire Police some weeks previously for a missing person. The present body had in fact been found in the Metropolitan Police area, but the Hertfordshire officers were naturally concerned as well. The two neighbouring forces had cooperated in searching the area around the railway station where the missing person – a 29-year-old secretary, Mrs Ann Lock, recently married and working at Thames Television – had last been seen. At 10 p.m. on Sunday 18 May she alighted at Brookmans Park station to collect her bicycle from an adjoining shed and cycle the short distance home. Her husband was away for the weekend on a short break.

The body discovered by the railway workers was that of Ann Lock all right. Her bicycle had been found the day after her disappearance, still locked, propped against a fence near the station. Later, some half a mile away, her telephone book and diary were also found. Taking into account the place where the body lay, it appeared likely she had been forced to walk along the railway path.

It was clear that extensive decomposition had occurred during the nine weeks since her death. Her clothing was still evident – a long-sleeved pullover, the front of which was distinctly marked by an area which had been burnt away, the margins of the material charred. A quilted anorak lay on her shoulders. The lower torso was not clothed; the jeans she had been wearing had been drawn down on to her lower thighs.

There were trainer shoes on her feet; the laces had been undone. Her socks were missing – a matter that was to form a very important part of the medical evidence. Her hands lay behind her body, with a length of tape still extant around a small fingerbone and the rest of the small hand bones lying adjacent in the decomposed tissue behind her body. The fingers of her right hand had been secured individually by that length of white tape, which had a distinctive seamed edge; it was looped at one end around the smallest bone of the little finger, and a series of knots were spaced inches apart in the material. There was a loop at the other end of the tape, too, but no bones were enclosed in either it or the knots.

The significant medical findings were in the skull, the bony outline of which was all that remained. One of Mrs Lock's socks was embedded in the back of the mouth cavity and the other was tied across the front of the lower jawbone, being secured at the back of the neck by a simple knot. There was evidence that, although the tissues of the face and skull had disappeared, the cause of death had been complete obstruction of her airway by the sock thrust to the back of the throat. I thought the position of the second sock across the lower jaw could be either because she had successfully resisted an attempt at strangulation by flexing her head, so the material could not reach her neck, or, alternatively, that the sock had been placed in that position to force her mouth open. It could scarcely have been tied initially between the upper and lower jaws as it would not have slipped from there to the position in which it was found.

Detectives thought her death was linked to two other rape-associated murders that had occurred within the previous year as well as to other cases of rape. The murders became known as the Railway Murders, owing to their occurrence in the proximity of the railway network around London.

Subsequently John Francis Duffy was arrested, and two years

later he stood trial at the Old Bailey on the counts of three murders and six previous rapes. Duffy, a slimly built man 5ft 4in tall, who had acquired an extensive knowledge and practice of martial arts, denied the charges, claiming amnesia. Such was the nature of the case that it aroused much public interest; when prosecuting counsel outlined the charges, the public gallery was full and the well of the court was packed with visitors and officials.

The prosecution case began with the first victim, a 19-year-old girl, Alison Day, who had travelled on the north London railway to meet her fiancé on 29 December 1985. As she left Hackney Wick station, east London, she was seized, taken a short distance, and raped by the side of a nearby canal. While she was being forcibly walked back from the scene of the rape she ran away, fell into the canal, managed to get out, and started to run again. She was caught once more and strangled by means of a distinctive tourniquet involving a piece of wood from an elderberry tree placed into the loop of the knot and tightened. She was then thrown into the canal, where her body was found some seventeen days later.

The second charge involved a 15-year-old schoolgirl, Martjee Tamboezer, who lived with her parents in Surrey. On 17 April 1986, while cycling along a path beside the railway line near her home, she was forced to stop by a piece of nylon cord stretched across the path. She was seized, taken to a field, knocked to the ground and raped, her hands tied together in front of her body by a long piece of string. Then, as she was being taken across another field, she was hit with a piece of rock, and fell unconscious to the ground. Thereafter she was strangled using a belt twisted around her neck, a piece of stick acting as a tourniquet in the knot. Next morning the body was found by some men hunting rabbits; of the three cases, her body was the only one to be found before decomposition had occurred.

My pathologist colleagues – Professor Peter Vanezis in the

case of Alison Day and Dr Roger Ainsworth in the second case – made detailed examinations and concluded that both deaths had been due to strangulation. The similarities between the three cases were more obvious with the first two murders. Clothing material was present in both victims' mouths, and a ligature and tourniquet had been used to cause strangulation and fracture the voicebox. Their knickers were missing, sperm was present, jeans were undone and shoes were missing or removed. The findings in the third case were not so similar, partly due to decomposition; however, although it was the sock in the mouth that had caused death, it appeared that there had been an attempt at strangulation.

Duffy was found guilty of the murders of the first two victims, but the judge directed the jury that there was a lack of evidence against him in the third case, that of Ann Lock.

I thought my involvement with the murder of Ann Lock had ended with a coroner's inquest in Watford the following year, 1989, when a verdict of unlawful killing was returned. And so the matter remained until the arrest of David Mulcahy in July 1998. He had been Duffy's soulmate since they had met at school in 1970. The arrest followed statements Duffy had made in prison to the forensic psychologist there, Dr Jenny Cutler. Duffy had by now been in prison for some ten years, and in 1997 he had been told that he would remain there for the rest of his natural life. Whether his statements were connected to guilt surfacing over the years or whether he thought his time in prison might be made more comfortable is uncertain; he may have realized that, if he were to spend the rest of his life in prison, there was no reason why Mulcahy should remain free, even though they had made a solemn pledge to each other long ago that, if one were arrested, the other would remain silent. He revealed to Dr Cutler that he had acted with his friend Mulcahy in some twenty-five sexual attacks on women, including three murders.

As Duffy's incrimination of Mulcahy would not be entirely satisfactory as evidence in a criminal trial, the crimes were once more put under scrutiny. Scientists found, by reference to a DNA database, that one of the original cases, involving the rape of a Danish au pair, showed evidence of Mulcahy's involvement. There had been insufficient evidence to incriminate him in previous rape cases and the three murders.

With the advancement of DNA techniques and following the breakthrough linking this single rape case to Duffy's submissions, detectives decided to charge Mulcahy, and a team of dedicated detectives, led by Superintendent Andy Murphy, pursued inquiries both in the United Kingdom and abroad, investigating and interviewing previous rape victims. Their efforts were a masterpiece of forensic investigation.

In September 2000 the case opened at Number One Court, Old Bailey, and, after several weeks of legal argument, the trial commenced. Ann Lock's murder had remained unsolved since the first trial, so it would be important in the second trial to test Duffy's allegation that Mulcahy had acted alone and was solely responsible for her death.

As we've seen, the mode of Ann Lock's death differed from the earlier two, where a tourniquet had been used to tighten the ligature around the neck; Mrs Lock's death, by contrast, was due to suffocation by the sock. This aspect of the case had been discussed at some length at a conference called by the prosecuting team led by Mark Dennis QC. It had been mentioned at the first trial, and we thought it could be an important point at the second, in that it showed a different *modus operandi* – a deliberate attempt by the assailant to force open the victim's mouth prior to placing the sock in it.

I gave my evidence relating to Ann Lock and my two colleagues gave evidence on the other murder cases – essentially the same evidence we had all given twelve years before. I had carefully examined the tape which had secured

Mrs Lock's hands, and I was cross-examined on exactly how the tape had been fastened to the fingers.

The trial lasted five months, the longest for a murder trial in the United Kingdom. On 12 February 2001 Mulcahy was found guilty of the three murders, seven rapes and five charges of conspiracy to rape. The judge described the crimes as acts of desolating wickedness, of violence that descended into the depths of depravity. Mulcahy was sentenced to a total of 250 years and three life sentences; he will spend the rest of his life in prison.

The case of two men being involved in a series of terrifying serial sex attacks and murders was unusual; as the pathologist for the defence pointed out in his report, serial killers are usually stereotyped as solitary persons who act entirely on their own.

Several of the rape victims who gave evidence faced aggressive cross-examination and strong suggestions that they were lying on behalf of the police. Nothing could have been further from the truth – as witnessed by their courage to come forward to be interviewed and give evidence.

The police investigation is not finished. There are still a considerable number of rapes and murders associated with rapes to be scrutinized in relation to their possible connection with Duffy's and Mulcahy's activities.

Chapter Two

Coroners' Quirks

The office of coroner is a very ancient and important one. In 1194 the Justices of Eyre were instructed to appoint 'custodians of pleas of the Crown' (*custos placitorum coronae*) in every county to generate revenue and to bypass the sheriffs. The powers included confiscation of a felon's property and included inquests on treasure trove and investigation of fires (no longer applicable). The office declined in the Middle Ages, but was revived in the nineteenth century with Acts of Parliament and further amendments of Coroners' Rules established later.

There are some two hundred coroners in the United Kingdom. The majority are outside the main cities, being solicitors who act as coroners on a part-time basis. By qualification a coroner must be a barrister, solicitor or registered medical practitioner of five years' standing, although coroners in London are usually dually qualified.

Basically, the coroner investigates all sudden unexpected natural deaths as well as unnatural and suspicious deaths reported to him or her. Although there is no precise legal definition of a doctor's duties in this respect, if the deceased's general medical practitioner has not seen the patient during the last illness, the GP should report the matter to the coroner. Doctors come directly into contact with coroners through reporting a death and through being summoned to give evidence or provide a report at an inquest in the coroner's court, which inquest is held if the death, following an autopsy, is found to have been unnatural.

In theory, detecting homicide is primarily the province of the pathologist, who is a key figure in the coroner's jurisdiction, performing autopsies at the coroner's request, supplying the coroner with a report of the findings, and giving evidence, if required, in court. The coroner has considerable powers, and is able to insist on an autopsy irrespective of the wishes of the deceased's family or of any religious objections. Until recent years, a pathologist would spend many hours in coroner's courts – a fact that provided excellent training for giving evidence and a first-class grounding for later appearances in a criminal court.

I worked for numerous coroners over the years, but the first was HM Coroner for the District of Middlesex (west of London). Previously he had for many years been a general practitioner in the poorer areas of north London. He ran his court at Ealing Town Hall three days a week, starting promptly at 9 o'clock. The pathologist had to attend to give evidence of the cause of death at the opening of an inquest, as well as subsequently to give his or her findings to all concerned. A jury was required to hear evidence and cases were completed within a few weeks of a fatality – rather than several months, as is the case now. I had never given evidence in a coroner's court before my appearances at Ealing Court, but he was sympathetic and indulgent of my efforts.

Another of the coroner's duties was to retain exhibits of knives and the like which had been responsible for a person's death. One morning he called me to his office. 'Bowen,' he said, 'do you remember that cut-throat suicide involving a carving knife, a few weeks ago?' Yes, I certainly did. 'Well,' he said, 'the knife and its accompanying cake slice made an excellent wedding present last weekend.'

He always required an officer in full uniform to apprise the court of his sitting. The officer in question had to hammer with his fist three times on the door leading to the court; those in court could sometimes see the panel move inwards, such was the vigour of the officer's fist blows. Once in court the officer had to announce the traditional opening of the court for proceedings to take place:

> Oyez, Oyez, Oyez. All manner of persons who have anything to do at this court before the Queen's Coroner for this County touching the death of *(name)*, draw near and give your attendance, and if anyone can give evidence, on behalf of our Sovereign Lady the Queen, when, how and by what means *(name)* came to his death, let him come forth, and he shall be heard.

A somewhat similar incantation was given at the end of the court:

> Oyez, Oyez, Oyez. All manner of persons who have had anything to do at this Court before the Queen's Coroner for this County touching the death of *(name)*, having discharged your duty, and you good men (and women) of the jury having returned your verdict, may depart hence and take your ease.

Proceedings were lengthy and on occasion, after a three-hour stint without interruption, the coroner would temporarily dismiss the jury – often a somewhat elderly bunch of men. They would leave the court in some haste with bowed heads, legs stiff as they went to obtain prompt relief in the gentlemen's cloakroom.

It was important that the jury consisted of not less than seven persons before the inquest commenced, and in a few jurisdictions it was sometimes difficult to issue subpoenas to jurors to attend. A pool was therefore formed of local worthies who were more than happy to stand in their stead. These people were almost professional jurors. On other occasions the mortician sometimes sat in court as a member of the jury. It was a custom which was soon abolished.

In the past the coroner's duty required him or her to see the body of the deceased if the death was the subject of an inquest. This was a tiresome procedure, particularly for the coroner's officer, as it quite often involved treks to outlying mortuaries that were a fair distance from the main court or the local police station, not to mention the chores involved in arranging for the coroner to attend the mortuary. On one occasion when the Ealing Coroner announced his intention to see the body, his officer realized with some panic that the deceased was already at the undertaker's chapel. Time was short. Being a resourceful officer, he risked his career and the wrath of his master by employing one of his colleagues to lie motionless and stone-like on the mortuary slab, covered with a shroud from the neck downwards. Fortunately the viewing went off satisfactorily.

Apart from the usual verdicts of accident, suicide and natural causes that a coroner can offer, there is the 'open' verdict. This is a curious but useful one as it indicates that, although the facts and findings of the case are evident, the circumstances surrounding the death are still not clear. It is particularly useful in deaths due to overdoses of drugs, where often the exact intention of the deceased is not clear.

After some years in Ealing I started to work for Dr Allan Cogswell, who was HM Coroner for the Northern District of London. The main court venue was in those days in one of the waiting rooms of the radiology department of a big north London hospital, as it was essential to provide somewhere convenient that relatives could reach easily. At one inquest the coroner explained to two elderly relatives of the deceased that I had given the cause of death as aspirin poisoning and he intended to return a verdict of suicide. Aspirin poisoning, uncommon nowadays, is extremely difficult to detect, not just because patients may not reveal their history of taking the tablets but also because the clinical signs may mimic other conditions. When the coroner's verdict was given in this instance, the deceased's elderly sister leapt to her feet to state that the deceased would never have taken her own life in this manner. Accordingly the coroner immediately quelled their fears and overturned his own verdict, saying he would now record the death as an accident. A jovial bon viveur, Cogswell would often ask me to join him for lunch at the pub after the inquest – an invitation I could scarcely refuse however inconvenient the timing. He was very much a coroner of the old guard.

After Cogswell retired I appeared for many years before his successor, Dr David Paul, who was in addition Coroner for the City of London, where I also worked with him. David Paul was a delightful person off the bench, but on it he was capable of causing mayhem among witnesses and great anxiety and stress in the court. He always got to the crux of, or found any weak point in, the evidence before him. Giving medical evidence was not too worrisome, as by the time one enters the witness box one has already ensured that nothing has been overlooked. But I saw many experienced police officers literally shaking while reading from their notes.

He was kindness itself to relatives, but not if provoked. One such occasion involved an overdose. The inquest had been adjourned for a week for the daughter of the deceased to attend court and give evidence. She arrived late for this second occasion, and was accompanied by her boyfriend. In magisterial tones the coroner questioned her as to why she was late, commenting that she had kept the court and, in particular, himself waiting. She explained she had overslept – she had been up during the night looking after her small children.

The boyfriend rose to his feet. 'Who are you?' the coroner boomed. 'I am her boyfriend, and I think you should get stuffed.' A stentorian 'Arrest that man!' rang out through the courtroom. The coroner has wide powers to detain, imprison and fine witnesses for contempt of court, and this was about to be demonstrated. The poor fellow was escorted to the coroner's room by the coroner's officer, and only by making the most abject of apologies did he escape being imprisoned or fined. As a souvenir I have the court tape-recording of this unusual event.

Medical witnesses and junior doctors were often a target for his tongue. I would sometimes wait for fireworks when a hospital doctor appeared dressed inappropriately, lacking jacket or tie – or, even worse, both – as I knew Dr Paul would pick on it: 'You have appeared before me dressed more in keeping with appearance on a tennis court than the coroner's court.' On one occasion, when a house physician said he did not actually possess such a thing as a jacket, I thought Dr Paul was going to order one of his officers to go to the hospital and search the man's wardrobe!

This coroner was very loyal to his staff, and always stood up for them against interference from an authority on the council or from uniformed members of the police force. The same went for his mortuary staff, in whose welfare he took a keen interest. He was greatly missed when he died prematurely – a martinet, perhaps, but a delightful character and a friend.

Coroner's officers play a unique role. In the old days they were police officers and thus naturally had a good working knowledge of the law, and of the ways of the general public. At one time the officers enjoyed not inconsiderable perks, and contacts with undertakers could be extremely valuable. In my early years witnesses were paid in cash. The sums involved were reckoned in guineas (a guinea was 21 shillings, or £1.05), and medical witnesses were expected to leave the odd shillings from their fees for the officers' benefit. In one court these transactions were performed near the exit door, and it always seemed incongruous that you could be discussing matters of life, death and bereavement to a background of the clinking of coins and *sotto voce* explanations to witnesses as to their monetary entitlements. With the increased stringencies on police-force budgets in recent years, coroner's officers are nowadays not serving policemen but civilians.

Mortuary staff are a heterogeneous group of men and, more recently, women. All must be fully trained and excellent at their work – the days of the untrained mortician have long gone. The aspiring mortician has to qualify for his or her position partly by apprenticeship but also by taking a Guild examination which provides a diploma in mortuary technology and hygiene. I had the privilege to work for many years with three talented men who were dedicated to their job and skilled in handling distraught relatives. Not all morticians were so sensitive. One whom I knew once telephoned the coroner to complain that he had insufficient work to cover his livelihood: could the coroner kindly arrange to send more bodies to his building? Another time I found a scrawled notice pinned to the door of a small, badly-equipped mortuary: 'Sorry, Sir. Cannot work in these conditions. Gone home.' I fully agreed with the man's views – the mortuary was attempting to deal with far too many cases with little assistance and few facilities – and so I reported the matter to the coroner.

The mortuary in north London I attended for some thirty-five years was attached to the coroner's court upstairs – advantageous, as I could be summoned at literally a moment's notice to give evidence.

On one occasion that I recall the pathologist, had he been summoned to leave the mortuary for the court, wouldn't have been able to make it . . . for the simple reason that he was staggering about the examination room – not from the effects of alcohol, I hasten to add, but due to exposure to a toxic solvent.

It was a bizarre occasion. The lecturer in the department, Dr John Butt, had been called as a matter of some urgency to examine the body of a middle-aged man who had collapsed in his garage. At the examination, Dr Butt found clear fluid in the man's stomach and, in the absence of evidence of natural disease, decided to collect and retain it for laboratory examination – which he did in the way that was usual in those days, pouring it into a perspex container and closing the jar. While writing out labels and attaching them, he noticed that the porcelain slab on which the jar rested was wet. So, taking a hot moist sponge, he quickly mopped the surface. The next thing he knew he was recovering consciousness. Fortunately the superintendent, who had been in another part of the building, returned to the mortuary to find Butt staggering around the room, and managed to prevent him from falling and hitting his head on the floor. He noticed an odd aromatic smell in the place, so guided Butt outside to the fresh air. Once Dr Butt had recovered, a reconstruction showed that the jar had partially dissolved, and that its contents had drained onto the porcelain surface. The fluid which Dr Butt had collected was chloroform, the deceased having taken his life by swallowing several ounces of fluid (from a metal container subsequently found on the garage floor). In dissolving the perspex jar the chloroform had released toxic vapour.

One never knows when a potential hazard may be encountered in one's work. The episode above reminds me of an occasion when I had been unable to find the cause of death of a person who had collapsed in a public house shortly after wishing the landlord goodnight. I had examined the man's clothing, and in a pocket of his overcoat had found a 10 oz medicine bottle labelled as a remedy for dyspepsia. Several ounces still remained. I wondered if there might be any possible connection between it and the man's demise, and showed it to the coroner's officer. 'Nothing to it, Doc,' he said. 'I'll just have a drop and see if it's similar to the medicine I'm taking for my stomach.' Fortunately I prevented him from doing so. The 'medicine' was, in fact, cyanide.

A little-known aspect of a coroner's duties concerned holding an inquest after a judicial execution, or hanging. When lecturing, if I ran out of medico-legal questions for the students I sometimes asked them in what circumstances a coroner's jury was summoned when the person on whom they were required to give a verdict was still alive. I was never given a correct answer.

In one such instance three youths – one being Victor John Terry, aged 20 – were tried for murdering a bank guard. The Crown's case was that Terry had deliberately shot the guard with intent to kill, having entered the bank with a loaded gun ready to fire. Terry was found guilty of murder at Sussex Assizes, and sentenced to death, being sent to Wandsworth Prison, south London.

I was instructed by the coroner to carry out the autopsy following the execution, in May 1961. In such cases the coroner had to hold an inquest immediately, subsequent to judicial execution, so required a jury to be selected several days beforehand. The all-male jury at Wandsworth was duly assembled, and my evidence following my examination showed the appearances of judicial hanging, with considerable separation between the second and third spinal bones at the base of the skull and severance of the spinal cord, the mark of a ligature on the neck much higher up than seen in suicidal hanging. As far as I was concerned I was glad it was over. The jury duly returned their verdict.

The last occasion a judicial execution took place in this country was on 13 August 1964, when two men found guilty of murder were hanged at the two different prisons where they had been held. A year later, in November 1965, Parliament decided to suspend capital punishment for a trial period. In December 1969 an Act of Parliament abolished capital punishment for all offences save treason.

Coroners' quirks may soon be an arcane phenomenon in this country judging by recent developments. There are two official enquiries in progress into the system – the Shipman Inquiry concerning the deaths of some 215 patients of Dr Harold Shipman, a general practitioner in Greater Manchester who poisoned many of his patients; also a Home Office enquiry into death certification and associated procedures, including the role of pathologists and coroners. The present system will be radically changed, possibly replaced by Medical Examiners as in the USA, leaving judicial enquiries relating to death in the hands of the remaining coroner set up.

Chapter Three

On Probation

After my initial six years in hospital pathology, life as a junior forensic pathologist was completely different – and very hectic, especially when compared with the more leisurely work I'd been accustomed to in the laboratory. I had no experience in medico-legal work, never having given evidence in coroner's court or any court of law, nor done any teaching. The new post I took up was as Demonstrator in Forensic Pathology at St George's Hospital Medical School.

Basically my work involved going to tumbledown Victorian mortuaries in northern and western Middlesex and doing cases which my chief decided he couldn't manage, chiefly because they would have involved his attendance at inquests. I could see that my future depended on my not making a hash of any cases; if I did, the coroner would dispense with my services. When I was not carrying out autopsies or testifying in coroner's court, I followed the master around his domain while he performed a formidable number of post-mortems daily. At one such mortuary in those early days, as he was preparing for work, he asked if I ever wore a stiff collar – my current collar was of the soft variety, and obviously not up to scratch. Thereafter I always wore a stiff white collar . . . although I found out later that his own stiff collars were of the paper variety!

There were three forensic departments in London at that time, all developed through the efforts of individual pathologists working initially for the London coroners and establishing links with the medical schools. The London Hospital Medical College had at one time a large department with some half-dozen part- and full-time pathologists who came and went according to the senior man's requirements. Francis Camps, its head, was an entrepreneur, and his staff were salaried. Camps had no formal training in general pathology but had been a bacteriologist and had worked in general practice. At Guy's Hospital Keith Simpson had already established his position as an outstanding medico-legalist and lecturer, and at St George's my chief, Donald Teare, a warm-hearted gentleman, completed the triumvirate.

These Three Musketeers, as they were known, coped with almost all the crime work, suspicious deaths and murders in the London area, so it was very difficult to get a foothold in that sphere. Almost all of my own work concerned natural deaths plus a fair number of unnatural ones, but not those deaths requiring CID involvement. My naivety in the new sphere was painfully obvious in an early case, where no crime was suspected. A prosperous barrister collapsed and died from a heart attack while at the house of a lady friend, and the coroner's officer mentioned that the deceased had been involved in a traffic accident. He either didn't know or inquire as to its nature, or was waiting to see the case unfold in the coroner's court; I suspect that he thought I was an obstruction to the pathologist for whom he provided most of the coroner's work in his area. A few months after commencing work, then, I was subjected to an hour-long cross-examination in court by the deceased's family's barrister.

It transpired that the deceased had sustained a number of fractures, was incapacitated and was still so at the time of death. Surely, the family's barrister plugged away, the injuries must have contributed in some way to the man's death. I refuted his views, but was aware that I was doing so stumblingly. It was all very unsatisfactory, and so it was obvious to me I had to enter a rapid learning curve – in future I should inquire into the background of any case.

I will never forget Kilburn mortuary in northwest London. With the coroner's court it could have been a listed building. In retrospect, it was a place which nowadays would be chosen as a scene for a television crime documentary. The approach was by way of a cobblestoned forecourt. Attached to the wall outside the small mortuary was a large glass case – rather like an open wardrobe – with hooks on which, in days gone by, the clothing of the deceased was hung so that relatives were spared the painful process of direct identification.

I had an unusual pathological investigation and one near-fatal disaster at this place. Working in the afternoon on a sudden death, I heard the rumble of the undertaker's hearse over the courtyard. One could almost picture a horse-drawn funeral carriage, as must have been the case in bygone years. The body was taken from the hearse to the tiny annexe, and shortly afterwards I heard a thunderous shout of: 'She's alive! Where's the doc?'

Hastily I laid down my instruments and entered the annexe. Solemn white-faced undertakers ringed the coffin. I noticed the 'deceased's' chest moving, and eventually established that the respiration rate was about eight breaths per minute. Obviously the patient had to be revived, which would best be done by enveloping her body in blankets to raise the core temperature – as clearly the underlying condition was hypothermia. This accomplished, I asked the undertakers to return her to the hearse and transport her back to the hospital. This proved a sticking point. Whether from some inborn fear or respect for the dead, the undertakers declined; they requested an ambulance. This was actually more sensible from a practical viewpoint, as ambulance staff could take further measures to breathe life into her body. Although the hypothermia appeared irreversible, I learnt later that she survived in hospital for some thirty-six hours, albeit unconscious.

No blame was attached to the casualty staff for the error; it is well recognized that such cases can occur in winter. Depending on the degree of drama involved, they usually warrant a small paragraph in the local paper or a larger one if some hospital authority or doctor is thought to have been responsible. In this instance it was ascertained that the woman had been found lying unconscious, due to a barbiturate overdose, on a cold stone floor. Barbiturate overdose was second only to carbon-monoxide poisoning as a cause of suicidal death in those days. Nowadays neither category of death occurs much, although there are sometimes cases of carbon-monoxide poisoning due to faulty central-heating units or in an enclosed car.

Taken to casualty, the woman had been seen and examined by two doctors, pronounced dead, and transferred to a refrigerated compartment in the mortuary. There the matter would have, quite literally, rested had it not been for the arrival of the undertakers who'd been called to take the body of another person to the local coroner's mortuary. Noticing that the woman's body next to the one they'd come for was a coroner's case, they'd helpfully decided to take both in their hearse.

I have no doubt that the doctors who examined her in casualty found the usual signs of death. Spending a short time in the hospital refrigerator and then being conveyed in the relative warmth of the hearse allowed her core body temperature to rise and respiration to become evident. The underlying condition, barbiturate poisoning, always depresses the respiratory centre of the brain and lowers body temperature.

A similar condition is encountered when the victim rapidly develops hypothermia following immersion in cold water, so in all such cases it is vitally important to persist with methods of warming and resuscitation.

Another unusual occurrence at that mortuary came a few years later. In those days Saturday-morning attendance at mortuaries was compulsory because the hard-pressed senior men wished to lessen the work that would accumulate over the weekend. The episode I refer to occurred on an Easter Saturday – it being essential over the Easter break to restore some degree of normality to the mortuary schedule. The mortuary staff comprised the superintendent, who was generally a cheery soul, and his assistant, who never responded to my usual greeting on arrival and, indeed, seldom uttered a word at all. In those days it was the practice also for the coroner's officer to attend the pathologist's visit, so that he could expedite the inquiries and, often, provide answers in matters relating to the history.

Noon was approaching and, as I did not wish to prolong my work, I spoke somewhat sharply to the assistant, instructing him to place shrouds on two cases so that they could be taken out to the annexe. I had turned away to attend to some specimen when my thoughts were interrupted by unusual growling sounds. As I turned back I saw the assistant taking one of the larger and presumably sharper mortuary knives and – eyes staring – gathering his relatively small frame to approach me. Thoughts of some swashbuckling dive across the mortuary table were not uppermost in my mind at that moment!

Luckily the coroner's officer saved my skin – although, from my assailant's demeanour, it was more than skin he had in mind. Despite his sixteen stone, the coroner's officer, a policeman of long standing who rejoiced in the name of Mr Boddy, strode between myself, the table and my adversary. In a short time the mortician was disarmed and escorted out of the building; the coroner was informed and the man was dismissed forthwith. Little regard or inquiry had been made by the employing authority as to his credentials; his application form merely stated that he had assisted in the recovery of bodies and examination of soldiers on fields of battle during the Second World War. Sadly, the gallant Mr Boddy collapsed and died some years later while attending a funeral.

The difficulties the subject could present if I didn't have a detailed history of the circumstances surrounding a final illness were indicated to me at an examination that I witnessed at this mortuary.

A middle-aged woman had been admitted to the local district hospital in a comatose state, with evidence of peripheral nerve disorder. After several days without diagnosis she died, and the doctors referred the death to the local coroner. The autopsy did not reveal any specific abnormality or disease and eventually, after examination of the spinal cord, a diagnosis was made of some softening of the substance due to a viral inflammatory disease. Her body was cremated.

Three years later her 15-year-old stepson, Graham Young, was found guilty at the Old Bailey of the attempted murder of his father, sister and friend. He received a ten-year sentence, served in Broadmoor, but was released before completing it. Subsequently, now twenty-three years of age, he obtained employment, his past record unnoticed, at a photographic-equipment laboratory in Hertfordshire. Some six months after that he fatally poisoned two colleagues with thallium – available in the laboratory. In June 1972 he was charged with the deaths of the two men and with two further attempted murders. This time he was sentenced to life imprisonment. He died of a heart attack in 1990.

In the 1960s there were no sophisticated techniques for drug analysis; nowadays his stepmother's death would be the subject of a complete analysis using chromatography and spectrophotometry.

Some time later a new assistant arrived at the mortuary to replace my would-be assassin. I sometimes thought the newcomer was blamed for everything that went wrong. One incident that was certainly his fault came to my notice early on a winter's morning when I arrived to start the day's work. The large porcelain mortuary table lay shattered in large chunks over the floor. The assistant, on his own that day, had placed the bodies of two people on the mortuary table, certainly not an approved practice. There must have been an uneven weight distribution because the table, with its single central pedestal, was not robust enough to support the combined weight, and snapped. The assistant was hobbling about with a bruised foot from one of the broken slabs.

The superintendent was always most helpful but, as my secretary noticed whenever I was there at the same time as my chief, Donald Teare (usually watching him work), my chief reduced the man to a nervous wreck, so that everything he did or said resulted in some form of reprimand – not always unamusing, bearing in mind the black humour that often exists in mortuaries.

An example was the disastrous loss of a valuable specimen that my chief had reserved. Coroners may authorize specimens to be retained, particularly for toxicology; but tissues, other than for matters relating to the cause of death, are not taken. It is also recognized that the interment of a body should be complete: relatives may insist that any organs removed are subsequently buried with the rest. In this particular case, the brain showed characteristic signs of anoxia due to loss of blood supply following barbiturate poisoning; as this is a very rare and unusual pathological entity, the plan was to preserve the specimen and place it in a medical museum for the use of the students.

Medical-school museums were probably more popular (or at least used) in the past than nowadays. It is generally recognized that the medical schools are entitled to their museums, although it was thought originally that the one at the Royal College of Surgeons was the only one to have been established legally.

Donald Teare indicated to the superintendent – who by this

time was as usual flushed, his demeanour agitated and his hands, unfortunately, shaking – to lift the brain with his fingers around the circumference. Unfortunately, the superintendent's thumbs pressed into it exactly in those areas where the unusual pathology existed, so destroying for all time its appearance and significance. For a moment there was a silence, then an explosion of wrath caused the mortician to drop the specimen on the floor.

That ancient building has long since been replaced by a housing estate. The fault of these small mortuaries lay in the fact that all the local authority had to provide was a building with minimal facilities, such as running water, in which the deceased could be kept until burial or cremation – particularly if they had collapsed in the street rather than in a hospital. These buildings were totally inadequate by present-day standards. The coroner's court attached was almost always, by contrast, well appointed, with rich mahogany benches/pews, a witness box and appropriate seating for the coroner, relatives, press and solicitors. Several such courts had, near the door, a polished collecting box with a brass inscription soliciting money for the coroner's charities.

I had more than my fair share of inquests as Donald Teare had insufficient time to attend some courts. I was interested in unusual cases, and was able to publish a number of papers, the most notable concerning a condition which, probably incorrectly, became known as Bowen's Disease! Whilst carrying out an autopsy on a stroke victim I discovered an appearance of the windpipe that I'd never encountered before: its lining had a cobblestoned look instead of a smooth surface. I took the specimen to the hospital, where it met with a mild degree of interest, one or two people suggesting the condition was an odd development of the air passages. Odd indeed. The Professor of Pathology, Theo Crawford, showed a greater curiosity, and eventually a paper was published. Although the condition had been recognized previously – there had been some ninety cases in all, world-wide, the most interesting being one reported by a Charing Cross Hospital physician in the 1850s – only a couple of instances had been recorded in the English-language literature. Thus the condition was denoted in the *American Medical Dictionary* as Bowen's Disease – or, to give it its full title, tracheo-bronchiopathia osteochondroplastica. I know this only because much later my son, as a medical student, came across it when he looked up 'Bowen' in his dictionary.

The specimen was eventually presented to Charing Cross Medical School Museum, where it stood next to a skull from a well known murder case. The latter was eventually stolen from the museum at the same time as a complete case of historical ENT (ear, nose and throat) instruments, presumably 'to order'.

A most unfortunate specimen with which I had to deal was one from an unsolved murder. It had lain in the preparation room at St George's Hospital for a year or so and, when inquiries into the case had been abandoned, it was obviously correct to dispose of it in a decent manner. Anticipating this event, I placed it on the surface of a low desk in the small, rather old-fashioned forensic department at St George's Hospital. The department was in two sections: the upper floor where the chief and secretary worked, and lower one, where I had a small desk (chiefly for my secretary) and the technician, in a little laboratory, had a rather larger desk. One evening before I left the department, I put this specimen on the technician's desk for him to deal with in the morning.

The department, certainly on the lower level, had a some-what gloomy appearance at the best of times, as there were no windows. The following morning, early, the cleaners arrived to do their usual chores. One was attending to the floor of the technician's laboratory and, when she straightened up, her gaze was level with his bench – and the specimen, a skull. With a cry of horror she fled. The other cleaners downed tools – or mops – and went to see their supervisor, who decided it must be a sick joke. When I got there at lunchtime, I had to explain that there was nothing untoward about the occurrence; I had had no idea of the cleaners' early-morning routine. I hastily denied any form of intended joke. Grudgingly, my explanation was accepted.

The three senior forensic pathologists – Camps, Simpson and Teare – were usually accompanied by their secretaries as they travelled to and fro across London working for the London coroners. I was advised to work in a similar manner, although my work quota was very small by comparison. The reason for this system of work was that in those days coroners required reports to be available the day of the examination. In later years pathologists could bring in reports dictated on to mini-recorders, but even so untyped case reports could soon pile up. I recall one departmental secretary in particular whose backlog of cases reached stupendous levels, much to the chagrin of the coroners and their officers.

Over the years I was blessed with excellent secretaries – three in all, over thirty-five years. Bear in mind that it was not a calling for the faint-hearted. The first worked part-time. Her successor, who was extremely efficient, journeyed up from the south coast daily. She enjoyed the hustle and bustle of going around the metropolis and out into the suburbs with me. As we were hurrying back to London one day in my open car, a number of copies of my reports flew out from the small back seat and scattered themselves along the roadside. Despite a plea from my secretary I drove on. I had no time to stop and retrieve them. I hope I didn't give some innocent countryman too frightful a shock.

Opportunities for investigating the medical aspects of homicide were almost nonexistent unless the chief was away, and any work in that sphere that did come through was as a result of being called in by coroner's officers. There is a curious relationship between the coroner, the coroner's officer, the pathologist and the CID. A pathologist working in a coroner's area will be asked to carry out examinations on deceased persons reported to his jurisdiction. If the death is suspicious, the pathologist will also be asked to carry out the autopsy; in addition, the death will automatically be reported to the CID, and a senior officer will attend the examination. The same procedure applies in a murder investigation, although those present at the autopsy will also include a scene-of-crime officer, a photographer and a laboratory liaison officer, the latter to deal with specimens or other forms of evidence collected and carefully itemized in sealed containers.

Should the coroner regard the pathologist as too inexperienced to deal with a murder, he or she will ask a more senior practitioner to carry out the autopsy. Indeed, years ago it was automatic for the senior pathologist to be the one called in for any murder. The symbiotic relationship between coroner and pathologist was very close in those times; it is much more open nowadays. The coroner can, of course, inform the pathologist at any time that he or she no longer wishes that individual to work in the coroner's jurisdiction.

The CID officers, for their part, were highly motivated and professional thanks to the system whereby the officers had risen through the ranks. The scene-of-crime officers had a vocation and profession for life – always at the scene of an incident, attending all examinations of suspicious deaths, and relying on the pathologist for the answers. One could sometimes almost see them listening to every word uttered on findings and opinions. Nowadays CID officers are expected to transfer to uniform duties as part of their career, so the practice has changed completely.

The haphazard nature of the system was illustrated by the fact that my big breakthrough came in another area of London entirely from the one in which I generally worked. There were two small jurisdictions in which I could find work other than the scraps that fell from my master's table. I had done a few inquest cases for the Coroner for the Northern District of London, Dr Arnold Piney, the principal pathologist for that area was the coroner's close friend. A cultured man with a distinctive black beret, which gave him a somewhat raffish appearance, he had written a book on haematology. He had no car, so relied on coroner's officers to pick him up for the journey to the mortuary and court building, which was attached to the main district hospital. His knowledge of pathology was sound, but in practice he relied on the mortuary superintendent to indicate to him the likely cause of death. He was getting on in years and knew that time was running out for him; accordingly, he let it be known that he wished to attend only two or three days a week. The remaining days fell to a colleague from another teaching hospital. After a few weeks, this colleague informed the coroner that it was clear the officers were keeping most of the cases for the days when the now semi-retired pathologist was available. He wasn't prepared to carry on working that way, so I got a call from the coroner asking me if I could help out. I did so. Within a month the old pathologist collapsed and died, and I was asked to take over the jurisdiction on a full-time basis. So, by pure happenstance, I'd arrived!

The work involved me in the investigation of suspicious deaths and homicide in a very large area of north London. No doubt I made mistakes, but my greatest fear was of forming a dogmatic opinion that would not stand up in court – unfair on the accused, and disastrous for the pathologist.

During this time I became increasingly concerned about the fact that death due to drug overdose was often suspected but impossible to prove scientifically. Indeed, I thought diagnosis in such instances was often little better than guesswork, apart from in cases of carbon monoxide poisoning and a rather crude method of analysis for alcohol. I therefore persuaded my chief, Donald Teare, to contact the laboratory at Scotland Yard so that I could attend and observe their investigation and laboratory analyses. In the 1960s toxicology was still in its infancy, of course; this was well before the advent of high-pressure liquid chromatography and mass spectrometry. The forensic laboratory at Scotland Yard dealt with all manner of suspicious poisonings around London, but not suicidal or accidental ones – the analyses being mainly of a chemical nature. I brought back information and access to basic instrumentation which our laboratory technician at St George's used to improve our analytical results.

At Charing Cross Hospital Medical School a pathologist who had developed an interest in forensics had a long-standing immune disease illness which ultimately caused his death. He also lectured to a small but enthusiastic group of students and, following his untimely demise, the Medical School advertised the post of part-time lecturer. I seized on the idea and, with the support of Teare and the local coroner, Gavin Thurston – who himself had been filling in as the Medical School lecturer – I applied for the post. It was characteristically generous of Thurston to act as he did; he was genuinely interested in the subject and eager that it should advance, and in particular he was keen on bringing on younger practitioners.

There were a couple of other candidates at the formal interview, and I was relieved when I heard I'd got the job. Officially the appointment meant a partial change of venue; luckily my secretary was willing to accompany me to Charing Cross.

I didn't know at the time that this would become a full-time occupation. Soon, though, I realized that I could not carry on at St George's. I therefore decided to cut the umbilical cord – much to the dismay of my chief, Donald Teare, who perhaps thought that by taking my share of the work with me I would undermine his department and possibly his territory. Nothing could have been further from my mind.

Chapter Four

The Deep End

After ten years' working experience, I could see I had the knowledge and ability to develop something worthwhile in my new position at Charing Cross Hospital Medical School. I had been warned that forensics was a sensitive subject there, as there had been unease among the pathology staff concerning the former pathologist, who had been doing part-time forensic work and had created minor jealousies, but in fact I saw no evidence of such feelings, and I was made welcome. My office was a tiny room on the first floor overlooking Agar Street – known colloquially as the Agar slope (as used in bacteriological culture media). The main building of the Medical School occupied an old Victorian development a stone's throw away from the famous hospital itself – a magnificent listed building with an historic background. My office had been little-used, as evidenced by the thick covering of dust when I arrived. A quaint upper floor was reached by a rickety stepladder and enclosed by some wooden railings of doubtful strength. The entrance and exit were also hazardous, with a narrow right-angled turn into the stairway opposite an ancient lift. My first assistant, becoming worried about the situation, attached a long coil of rope to the radiator next to the only window that overlooked the street so he could abseil down in the case of fire!

I had the good fortune that I was supported from the outset by the senior histopathologist, Professor W. S. St. C. Symmers, an eminent man appointed most exceptionally in his early thirties who had already written a standard textbook on the subject and some other outstanding books on pathology. His hours of attendance were unusual: late afternoon to midnight, seldom seeing his secretary or members of staff, and so immune from face-to-face discussion with the latter. I wondered how it would pan out. The Medical School secretary was a gregarious man, full of enthusiasm for forensic work in the school and willing to help those consultants whom he thought genuine.

I had no salary at the time, so I decided I could only advance my station and subject by funding certain things myself. I had a small signboard I'd brought with me from St George's Hospital that said 'Department of Forensic Medicine', so I nailed it to the entrance door. Some senior staff members were outraged by this – there was no mandate for a department whatsoever – but others were amused and the school's secretary was delighted: it indicated future development.

The Medical School's small mortuary was usually full of students, all the more so whenever I dealt with a drug-addict death, something very uncommon at that time. Such cases were examined in the hospital by permission of the local coroner. There was a peculiar arrangement for transportation of a deceased's body from the hospital to the mortuary, which was on the top floor of the Medical School. In order that the deceased did not become a matter of public interest – as would obviously have been the case had the body been simply carried up the street in full view – there was a system whereby the corpse was placed on a stretcher in the bowels of the hospital and drawn on a sledge-like apparatus through an ancient tunnel beneath the road to the basement of the Medical School, where it was placed in a special lift to transport it to the topmost floor and mortuary facility.

One embarrassing event – and with hindsight it's surprising this didn't occur more often – concerned the examination of a person belonging to a religious sect that ordained burial within a day of death. The lift apparatus had broken down and so the body could not be transported in the usual way. While the coroner's officer for Westminster was occupied placating distressed relatives, the superintendent and his staff were frantically attempting to release the mechanism and complete their duties. Luckily they succeeded in the end.

On another occasion, while I was demonstrating (with, I admit it, a touch of theatre) a case of cyanide poisoning to a packed audience, I warned the students of the danger of missing the smell of cyanide, illustrating my point with references to cases from the past. Just then a student collapsed like a log to the floor, unconscious. I was horrified. Was he the victim of inhaling some cyanide vapour from the jar of fluid at my elbow? He had been quite close to the pot, and some people are incapable of perceiving the characteristic smell of cyanide – which normally, owing to its pungency, causes people reflexively to back away. I rushed to his side and made sure he was dragged out into the fresh air. All sorts of dreadful thoughts flashed through my mind – newspaper headlines: 'PATHOLOGIST KILLS STUDENT IN DEMONSTRATION OF CYANIDE POISONING.' Fortunately he made a rapid recovery – it had been a simple faint, the sort we all have on occasions when perceiving the idea in the back of our mind.

I was completely on my own now regarding toxicological examinations, as the resources of St George's were no longer available, so it became essential to get some sort of service started. Alcohol estimations were no problem, although they had to be set up, chiefly by my secretary, after the day's work had been completed. I purchased a second-hand spectro-photometer, a very crude-looking machine, for the estimations of barbiturates. I would prepare the extraction while my secretary fed the sample into the machine and, hopefully, we calculated the correct result. I soon realized I would have to employ a technician to take the work off our shoulders, and so I took one on part-time. He worked upstairs on the somewhat rickety platform.

I noticed the Medical School's secretary was wondering when I was going to expand my unit and employ an assistant to share some of the workload. Obviously it would mean a drop in my income, but the problem would have to be faced sooner or later. At Guy's Keith Simpson had a large number of peripatetic young forensic doctors in his department, chiefly from abroad, and, after discussing the matter with him over lunch, I more or less agreed to take on one of his supernumeraries. Nevertheless, by the time I left him I still hadn't made a final decision. He was keen to clinch the matter, though, and as I descended the open lift in the Guy's Medical School he shouted after me, 'Bowen, take my man.' Of course, I did. My new assistant, John Butt, proved to be an excellent pathologist, ambitious and hard-working, and with a zany sense of humour. After his time with me at Charing Cross Hospital he eventually, on obtaining a higher qualification, returned to Canada, where he became a respected medical examiner.

The one cloud on the horizon concerned my health. I was experiencing occasional sweats at night, was losing some weight and had a dry cough. It couldn't have been more plain to a bystander what was going on, but I had not myself, as is often the case with medical men, noticed anything much amiss as to its nature. I submitted to a chest X-ray – probably overdue anyway, because pathologists are supposed to have them at regular intervals. The radiologist, Seymour Reynolds, was a man who displayed a wonderful sense of humour in his habit of lightly touching on but not criticizing his colleagues' foibles. (I got to know him better when he became Dean of the Medical

School and I myself the Vice-Dean.) He looked at me and asked for a tomogram – a special set of X-rays to produce an image of varying depths of lung structure. It was clear from the tomogram that I had an active tuberculous lesion in my right upper lobe. This could have brought my career to a halt, at least temporarily. I was ordered injections of streptomycin, a powerful antituberculus substance never given for more than a few weeks owing to the development of resistance. (Two other drugs have been developed more recently that largely take its place.)

The Medical School microbiologist, when the matter filtered through to his department, requested a spit test from me to check for organisms. I took the two containers the bacteriology department gave me and, as I was going to Suffolk for the weekend, decided to produce the samples right away. Unfortunately, I couldn't drum up sufficient spit (sputum), so I added some drops of cold water from the kitchen tap, which hadn't been used for several weeks. Much to my surprise, the tests turned out positive and our well meaning microbiologist sought to suspend me completely from all duties! Luckily the Professor of Pathology did not cooperate, and much to the microbiologist's chagrin I continued at work. (The positive TB test on my sputum was probably the result of organisms akin to tubercle gathering in the water-tap. This was not a matter I could put to the microbiologist who, already fuming on my continuing at work, would not take kindly to my suggestion that his staining technique was not satisfactory.)

By this time I was on full chemotherapy. In due course the lesion became noninfective, and eventually it cleared. I suppose what had stirred the wretched TB organism into activity was my all-work-no-play lifestyle. Pathologists have always been the target for infections, and over the years a not inconsiderable number of them, especially before the antibiotic era, have developed life-threatening infections or even died following a minor cut or abrasion sustained during autopsies. One has only to inquire in the records of pathologists at other hospitals to confirm this view.

Things progressed at the Medical School. A growing concern was drug addiction, which had emerged as a serious problem although as yet nothing like the horror it became in subsequent years. In 1968 and 1971 regulations and acts of Parliament prohibited doctors from supplying drugs to addicts and controlled the misuse of addictive drugs. In one case it was recorded that an aged doctor had been writing prescriptions for his addicted patients from the back of a van. The onus was on hospitals to monitor and control the situation through the creation of drug-dependence clinics. Expert psychiatrists were appointed to look after the clinics. At Charing Cross Hospital we were very fortunate to have a remarkably well balanced psychiatrist, Dr Gillian Oppenheim, in charge.

One aspect of the work required an assessment as to whether a patient was actually an addict: some addicts attempted to conceal their addiction, while at the other end of the spectrum there were patients whose aim was to obtain drugs for their own use or to sell. Apart from a basic medical examination, proof of addiction depended on laboratory tests. Due to my previous exposure to Scotland Yard laboratories, I had an interest in and some knowledge of toxicology, and from my clinical-pathology days I was keenly interested in the results of laboratory investigations to prove a diagnosis. Addicts who attended the clinic at Charing Cross Hospital were tested for basic narcotic drugs – a relatively simple procedure even with our minimal resources.

There was talk of a large dependency laboratory being established at another hospital, and they put out feelers to the Charing Cross administration regarding a takeover bid for our service. When I heard of this intrusion I rang the hospital administrator and, in no uncertain terms, told him to 'get off his backside and do something to support our work'. He got off said backside and the threat evaporated, and the following year at a conference in New York on drug abuse I had the honour to give a brief account of our work and findings.

Looking back on our methods, they were crude by today's sophisticated standards, but our relations with the drug-dependency clinic were remarkably secure. From time to time we did have problem cases, but these were amicably discussed, and any divergence between clinical results and laboratory findings was ironed out. Happily this was the basis and formation of a first-class toxicology department which provided, apart from forensic analysis, a full drug-addiction screening service and therapeutic monitoring of drugs used in clinical procedures, including anti-convulsants, some psychiatric drugs whose levels required monitoring, and cardiac drugs.

The new Charing Cross Hospital and Medical School in Fulham was opened in 1973 and, naturally enough, offered an environment totally unlike the quaint ancient buildings in the Strand. The forensic department included a large main laboratory office and a lecturer's room, and it became essential to recruit more staff to do justice to the space allocated and to operate the state-of-the-art technology with which we equipped the place. Eventually there were four pathologists, two secretaries, a histology technician and some six toxicologists.

We had made our mark.

Chapter Five

Acting for the Defence

A pathologist appearing in a trial on behalf of the accused is not a new phenomenon, but in the past twenty years or so it has become a *sine qua non* in any criminal trial, so much so that coroners are reluctant to release a body for burial or cremation unless they have written agreement from the defendant's solicitors. It is now normal practice for a second autopsy to be carried out on any murder victim. Curiously, these examinations are said to be carried out by an 'independent' pathologist, although in reality he or she is working entirely on behalf of the defence. If there is more than one defendant, it is an entitlement that several pathologists be called to examine the deceased's body and give an opinion. By the time the third or even fourth pathologist arrives on the scene, the findings are usually somewhat compromised – not just by the passage of time but by the activities of the preceding pathologists. A few coroners disagree with this procedure, and are quite prepared to ease the deceased's family's bereavement by allowing earlier reclamation of the body.

The cult of second examinations came into prominence in the 1970s and 1980s. Sometimes the examination revealed more than anyone expected. A remarkable case occurred on one occasion when a second pathologist was asked to give his opinion as to the time of death – a vital matter in a murder, as the accused was alleged to have an alibi to cover the period involved. The photographs made available from the initial investigation revealed that the fatal injury had been a firearm wound and not, as originally reported, a blow from a blunt instrument. The outcome was that an exhumation was ordered. The firearm wound was confirmed, and the case came to a halt because of the entirely different cause of death given originally.

The downside of defence work is that one can become tied to the defence solicitor's apron strings – he or she can ask you to attend case conferences and appear at the magistrates' court or crown court and spend the best part of the day listening to evidence.

When doctors or clinicians are called to give evidence following their examination, their fees are usually paid through the Legal Aid system and are not infrequently larger than those received by the pathologist who made the examination on behalf of the coroner and police authority. Indeed, until the 1980s only one fee was payable – and that from coroner's disbursements as, in the Metropolitan Police area at least, no additional payment was made for a pathologist's report in a suspicious death or murder inquiry. This state of affairs grew from the view that the pathologist was employed by the coroner and that his report went to the police through the coroner's courtesy.

The standing of forensic pathologists was eventually rationalized by a Home Office Working Party, whose findings were generally accepted and adopted in 1990. This was the latest of several attempts to give credence to and provide a career structure in forensic pathology. It ensured the financial stability of departments in London as it prescribed a contract between the Metropolitan Police and the relevant medical school, granting the latter substantial fees from its pathologists' work. Medical schools were thus able to retain their departments without having to draw on university or medical school funds for that purpose. In fact, this no longer pertains in London because the medical schools have, for academic reasons, decided to close their departments; only one forensic subdepartment remains.

Defence advice is sometimes sought on an informal basis, as when a colleague consulted me about a relative of his through marriage who had been found guilty of poisoning his wife and given a life sentence. The wife's death had been the subject of an autopsy by a hospital pathologist, and no forensic pathologist had been involved at any time, nor had a medico-legal opinion been sought. This mistake had been realized after the trial had finished, and now efforts were under way to find medical evidence which could reverse the decision of the court. I assisted as far as possible, although I could not see how the previous findings could be refuted; they seemed perfectly valid to me. Nevertheless, the case showed the importance of obtaining an opinion prior to trial. Recently Lord Wolff's report laid down that the prosecution's expert medical witnesses must be objective, must supply the court with their opinion beforehand, and must share it with the defence experts – somewhat as in the Scandinavian system.

A typical defence case concerned the death of a young lad, Mark Berkshire, aged 11, whose body was found concealed on waste ground fully clothed but with the trouser zip undone. Decomposition was considerably advanced, suggesting death some two months previously, in keeping with when he had been reported missing, and so there were no internal organs present.

Leaving other findings aside, the skin from the left side of the neck of the victim was examined, photographed and preserved. It is known that, if skin is exposed to ultraviolet light, it may reveal a pattern of bruise discoloration that can give more precise information as to the time the bruise occurred or may reveal underlying bruising. Carrying this test out on decomposed skin is not ideal – in my opinion its value is doubtful.

The pathologist, Professor Keith Mant, carried out the postmortem in November 1978, using this technique as well as infrared lighting and photography. He identified a rectangular mark on the skin in a position one might find in a case of strangulation. This area extended from the region of the left shoulder at the base of the skull and lower jaw, and was about half an inch long and a quarter of an inch wide. The skin differed here from elsewhere, and this was thought to be consistent with the application of a tight ligature, particularly as some chafing of the outer skin layers was visible under the microscope. The cause of death was therefore given as ligature strangulation. Professor Mant maintained in court that the mark on the skin, although it was impossible to say if it had been made before or after death, was consistent with that produced by a ligature, and that death could have been due to asphyxia.

A lengthy cross-examination ensued when I appeared as a defence witness. It is sometimes difficult for the stenographer to understand medical witnesses' evidence being taken down as transcripts for the court. An example of this occurred when the court transcript referred to Mant's description of 'vaginal inhibition' instead of 'vagal inhibition' – the latter being the sudden death of a person following light pressure on the neck when that victim is in a highly excited or frightened state. Death by vagal inhibition is due to the reflex arrest of the heart by stimulation of a nerve in the neck which has some control over the heart's pumping action. It was conceded in court that a number of causes of death were possible, although natural death in a boy of this age would be highly unusual.

The role of the open zip fastener on the boy's clothing was explored. The fact that it was undone, including the top button, without disturbance of the trousers might indicate that the unzipping had been carried out by someone prior to a sexual assault. I had appeared at the juvenile court and had suggested there were other possible explanations – that Mark might have unzipped his own fly to perform a natural function, that a dog might have tugged at the zip after death, or possibly that the process of decomposition had affected the clothing.

Moreover, reverting to the preserved skin specimen, if the neck had been subject to a ligature, a greater area of skin should have been affected, with more chafing of its surface. In all, it was impossible to place any firm significance on the mark, and I regarded the cause of death as unascertained.

The legal aspects of this case were interesting, as normally the prosecution is not allowed to produce evidence of a defendant's previous criminal conviction unless they can show, as alleged here, a striking similarity between the previous case and the case under consideration. (This is a very brief summary of a complex point of law.) It so happened that the accused had been convicted of assaulting a boy a year previously; the victim had said he felt something around his neck and had lost consciousness; when he later recovered, a piece of washing line had been found in the vicinity of the attack. The previous case was there- fore evidently one of attempted ligature strangulation so that, if the cause of Mark Berkshire's death could be shown to have likewise been ligature strangulation, such evidence could, arguably, be admissible to the court. It was curious how specifically the cause of death had been given, excluding all other possible causes; presumably the prosecution hoped, by focusing to exclusion on ligature strangulation, to be permitted to introduce the previous case as evidence. The defence accordingly challenged the right of the prosecution to refer to it. The judge, after studying previous law reports on the matter, said he had to rule in favour of the defence's argument.

From the juvenile court the case went to the Central Criminal Court, where the accused, a 17-year-old boy, was found guilty and sentenced to be detained indefinitely. It was only after the verdict had been pronounced that the previous conviction was read to the court. I heard later that the Director of Public Prosecutions had taken an inordinately long time to bring the case to court – some eighteen months – which suggests he had doubts about it going ahead.

In my summons to attend court it had stated categorically that I was 'not to depart the court without leave'. This arose because I was required that morning also to give evidence at the coroner's court in north London. The coroner had insisted that I should be at his court rather than the crown court, chiefly on the premise that the Number One Court at the Old Bailey had lesser precedence than the coroner's court. This point used to have significance; nowadays nobody is seriously concerned about it. In the end common sense prevailed and I was at the Old Bailey on time.

On another occasion an attempt was made to serve me with a similar summons, known as a subpoena ad testificandum, while I was at the department in St George's Hospital. The entrance to the main office was from the hospital corridor, and my secretary's desk was rather hidden at the end of the main office and reached by a short flight of steps (there being an exit door at the far end, down flagstone steps towards the mortuary). The summons said I was required to attend court to give evidence in a hearing concerning a fatal traffic accident. The laboratory technician, the secretary and myself played ducks and drakes for a while with the bearer of this missive – if he arrived while I was in the department I would, on receipt of a signal, hotfoot it through the exit. After several thwarted efforts he gave up his fruitless errand. I cannot recall what happened subsequently.

The only other time this sort of thing went on I was cunningly caught. I had received notice of civil case proceedings which I did not take seriously, and so I left it to the solicitor to contact me. However, my secretary had spoken to the firm and informed them that my attendance could be difficult, as I was going on a professional visit to Jordan. I arrived in the early evening at Heathrow Airport and was checking in when a young man tapped me on the shoulder and presented me with the subpoena document. He had taken pains to find out the flight times to Jordan, and had been tipped off by the clerk at the desk as to who I was.

The subpoena is a rather archaic procedure to ensure a witness's attendance at court, as nonattendance can result in a charge of contempt of court if the subpoena has been successfully served.

In court it is vitally important to present one's findings in layman's language, and to do so impartially, whether called by prosecution or by defence. There is no such thing as a run-of-the-mill court appearance for a medical witness. It may involve a short half-hour appearance or require giving evidence for a day. When multiple defendants are present on a murder charge, each will have a barrister appearing on their behalf, and the witness will have to deal with different questions from each barrister. Medical witnesses should not suppose they have the power or knowledge to prove the case for the defence or prosecution; it is a sad reflection on the personality of the witness if that is the attitude, and it smacks of megalomania. Looking round at the court, at the judge and the jury in particular, it is obvious they listen to the whole evidence and not just to the opinions of one ego-inflated doctor.

I remember an instance when a senior colleague, an exuberant and raffish rascal who had once attempted to monopolize forensic investigation and crime investigation in the capital, was engaged by the defence in a case concerning a young girl who had been found dead, fully clothed, on a mattress in a flat in north London. I had carried out the autopsy, and found an injection mark on her arm. The CID thought she had been the victim of an injection by an acquaintance rather than having administered it herself. Drug analysis was negative, examination of the tissues more informative.

Under the microscope the lungs showed an unusual reaction in the cells, rather like an inflammatory state but in fact due to the reaction of the tissues to the injection of a drug. An article in a US journal backed up my theory that, although this reaction did resemble pneumonia, the appearances were specifically related to drugs. I wrote to the author, an eminent New York forensic expert, Milton Helpern, to confirm his findings, but had received no reply, so, by the time of the trial for manslaughter of the young man accused of supplying and administering heroin to the girl, I was entirely on my own in the matter.

Having given my evidence, I was later recalled to the witness box when the aforementioned defence pathologist was giving his own evidence. I had previously lent him the microscope slides, but it came as a complete surprise when I returned to court to see large photographic blow-ups of the lung sections which my adversary – and I can use no other term cordially – was claiming confidently to the court showed signs characteristic of nothing but an early pneumonia, not drugs. The pictorial evidence convinced the court, but I knew the conclusion to be false.

I heard later that the defendant had subsequently been charged with possessing and supplying drugs and, appearing before the same judge, was given a substantial sentence.

On a lighter note, in another case at the Old Bailey I went to listen to the evidence of a colleague, Professor Keith Mant, in a case of stabbing. My brief was to give an opinion as to how it had occurred.

A pathologist giving an opinion to defending solicitors in a stabbing case has to deal with many aspects of the alleged assault. When it concerns a single stab wound, it opens up a line of inquiry which is sometimes exploited in court, the idea being that the accused did not purposefully stab the victim but that the victim might have fallen or run onto the knife, so turning the charge from murder to manslaughter – passive stabbing. It must be admitted that it is sometimes difficult to ascertain the exact sequence of events in a hand-to-hand skirmish, and all aspects of the wound must be taken into consideration – measured, compared with the width and dimensions of the knife submitted, or another knife, as well as respective heights of the victim and assailant. Evidence of an upward thrust into the chest is highly unlikely to indicate a running-on injury. So-called defensive or protective wounds – such as slashes on the forearm from trying to ward off a blow or on the hand from attempting to grasp the knife – are important as they indicate, to some extent, the direction of the assault.

Mant, a broad-shouldered man, was shown a large carving knife. Asked if he would examine it, he was offered latex gloves, an offer which he declined. In dramatic fashion he showed, beyond any shadow of doubt, how in his view the fatal wound had occurred. He raised his arm above his head, and a shaft of light from the court window glinted and flashed on the blade as he brought it down to chest level to indicate how the fatal injury had taken place. There was a cry from a lady in the front row of the jury box, and she collapsed in a heap on the floor.

I had no opportunity that day, or the expertise, to match Mant's histrionics. The court was adjourned and I was summoned by the judge to the jury room to administer first aid. I could find no palpable pulse, and at first I thought the worst had occurred. Could Mant have been indirectly responsible for an ischaemic heart attack? Fortunately, after medical aid, the jurywoman sat up and recovered completely.

There was nothing to contradict Mant's evidence and so the court – now minus one jury member, and with agreement from the accused man – continued with the case, which resulted in a guilty verdict.

Occasionally a seemingly straightforward case may cause the pathologist an unpleasant surprise – not the high-profile cases, where after numerous case conferences all matters have been thrashed out in advance. I recall in particular another stabbing trial, this time involving a single wound. I had given evidence in a straightforward manner in the morning, and had returned to the department – only to receive an urgent call for re-attendance at court that afternoon, where a master of oratory, Sir Ivan Lawrence QC, cross-examined me concerning the deceased's shirt.

Before the laboratory had tested it, I had examined the garment, as was my practice, and measured the slit in the material. Lawrence maintained that, as the length of the cut in the dry material was shorter than the width of the knife-blade alleged to have been responsible, it was therefore obvious that the cut had not been produced by the knife found in the accused's possession. The truth of the matter was that the victim had been stabbed while out of doors when it was raining; the shirt had dried and the cut in the material had therefore shrunk. Lawrence was making an unsuccessful attempt to draw attention to a small penknife which had been produced, and which was not the property of the accused. The defendant was subsequently found guilty.

A forensic pathologist is required to be acquainted with all aspects and complications of wounds and, occasionally, advice is required by Crown or defence that relies on the pathologist's specific experience in a particular field. Nowadays, with specialization in every branch of medicine, specialists are often called in on matters of forensic complexity. Head injuries, in particular, require an opinion from a neuropathologist.

One straightforward case where I assisted the defence did not in fact require such specialist expertise, although it was a most unusual complication of a stab wound and one that could hardly have been medically foreseen. A man and a woman were taken to hospital following a domestic affray. Apparently the man was accustomed to returning home the worse for drink, and had threatened his wife with a knife. She had responded by taking another knife and stabbing him in the neck. The woman had sustained a minor cut; the man, who had been found lying on the floor, had received a cut to the side of his neck, above his collarbone, and this was closed with sutures at the hospital. He was discharged the following morning, some seven hours later, and walked unaided to the ambulance. He had been told to return if there was any further bleeding from the wound. In the event, five hours later, he was brought in dead.

When the police arrived at the deceased's house a little before this to take a statement on the matter they had found the wounded man apparently asleep; on further examination they discovered he was moribund. The stitches of the neck wound were loose.

The man's wound, although superficial externally, had in fact penetrated an underlying vein, and his death was due to air having entered the circulation. There is a negative pressure in the neck veins if the person is standing or semi-kneeling, with the effect that air is sucked into the general circulation. This had not occurred at the time of the wounding because tissue swelling had sealed off the hole, and later the sutures had closed the skin wound. Only a sudden movement, such as coughing, could reopen the wound and stitches, and this is what had happened. The woman, who admitted the assault, was given a suspended sentence for manslaughter.

The condition of air embolism is a very rare event following a wound or a surgical procedure, and the only other case I have examined concerned a taxi driver who was punched in the jaw, resulting in a fracture. The following day, while under corrective surgery in theatre, he collapsed due to air entering a vein at the fracture site and hence the circulation – rare enough to warrant a case report in a medico-legal journal.

Air embolism was the most common cause of death in illegal abortions, usually at the hands of back-street abortionists. When the pregnant woman collapsed suddenly during the procedure, what often happened was that the body was quickly removed from the abortionist's house and dumped somewhere. Forensic pathologists like myself dealt with many such cases prior to the Abortion Act of 1967, after which they virtually ceased.

These deaths occurred because a syringe or instrument was passed into the uterus and then antiseptic fluid pumped into the cavity via an enema syringe, with the frequent result that a mass of churned-up air and fluid entered the uterus and hence the circulation, causing death instantaneously – much to the horror of the abortionist, of course. There were also a few cases in which the collapse was delayed until some hours after the abortion.

Occasionally high-profile cases turned up. One such was handed to me by Donald Teare, who asked me to contact solicitors engaged in defending a man on a murder charge, due to be heard at Gloucester Assizes. (The case has been documented by Professor Keith Simpson in his book *Forty Years of Murder*.) It was a most unusual affair, particularly as it hinged on difficult vital questions concerning the time of death of a man found decomposing (on 28 June 1964) in a Berkshire lane some hundred miles from his home. Quintin Hogg QC was appearing for the defence in his first criminal case since returning to the bar in May 1965; at the end of the first day of the trial he had to dash to London to take part in a division on the rising prices debate. Prosecuting counsel was Ralph Cusack QC, who outlined the case for the Crown, that Francis Brittle had murdered Peter Thomas, put him in the boot of a car, driven him from Gloucester to Bracknell, and there buried him in some woods – all because, so the prosecution maintained, Brittle had been unable to repay a loan of £2,000 made to him by Thomas and, becoming desperate, had decided to murder his creditor.

Brittle maintained that he had in fact repaid Thomas, using money won betting, but the prosecution had found no evidence of this. He was charged with murder following a coroner's warrant at an inquest – an unusual occurrence. The charge of murder is usually made following an appearance in a magistrates' court, and the fact that it had not been suggested the prosecution was not confident of the case.

A crucial piece of evidence for the defendant was that three witnesses maintained they had seen the deceased several days after the day on which the prosecution said he had been murdered. The first witness said he had seen Thomas on 20 June, the second that Thomas had been walking along the road near Blakeney on 21 June. Even more significant was the evidence of the third witness, a Mrs Padwick, who had served Thomas, a regular customer, in her shop on 21 June. Their evidence, despite numerous questions from Cusack, was not shaken.

In court it was stated that on 16 June, while driving from Gloucester to Bracknell, presumably with Thomas's body in the boot of the car, Brittle had given a lift to a golf caddy. The caddy had put his clubs in the car rather than the boot, perhaps at Brittle's suggestion.

Brittle himself was not called to give evidence. He had made contradictory statements to the police, and perhaps Hogg thought he would be open to lengthy and destructive cross-examination in the witness box.

Thomas, the deceased, had lived in squalor but had £4,500 in the bank at the time he met Brittle. He made the loan so that the latter could procure the lease on some gardens on the Earl of Radnor's estate near Salisbury and start up kennels. Brittle had no previous convictions for violence, but he had been discharged from the Army as medically unfit and for falsely claiming to be an officer. That record of Army service may have had some bearing on the manner in which Thomas had died, which was from a blow across the neck.

The body had been discovered on 28 June by a couple of lads looking for maggots prior to a fishing expedition. Simpson went to the scene the same day and formed the view, based entirely on observations made at the time, that death had occurred some 11–12 days before his examination. Specimens of maggots were retained for examination.

There was a pool of blood over the outside of the voicebox, and the small bones of the voicebox on one side of the neck had been broken. There was blood in the windpipe. All of this was in keeping with a blow to the throat causing haemorrhage around and into the air passages, and hence asphyxiation.

My view, after visiting Simpson, examining the tissues and taking pieces for microscopic examination, was that death had indeed probably occurred following a blow to the throat, although, curiously enough, the exact method of infliction was hardly mentioned at the trial; certainly not in the transcript of evidence. A karate- or commando-type blow to cause this injury is a horizontal chop with the extended outer side of the hand against the unsuspecting victim's neck; the victim immediately falls to the ground unconscious or dead.

The best-known example of this type of fatality occurred in the famous Emmett-Dunne case. A Regimental Sergeant-Major was found suspended in an Army barracks in Duisberg, Germany, in 1953, and the court of inquiry returned a verdict of suicide. At autopsy the initial findings were carefully and painstakingly recorded by the Royal Army Medical Corps pathologist: a fracture across the main cartilage of the larynx close to the thyroid gland. Unfortunately the Army pathologist had never previously examined a death due to hanging, and could not have been expected to recognize what had really occurred. In re-examination of the body by Francis Camps some time later, the injury to the larynx was found to have been due to a direct blow across the front of the neck. Evidence at the new hearing that this was indeed what had happened was given by the person who had assisted the accused, Emmett-Dunne, to suspend the body from the staircase banisters. Emmett-Dunne was convicted of murder at a General Court Martial in 1955.

In the case of R. v. Brittle, I had indicated to the defence team that, if they were to make any headway, they required the expertise of an entomologist – an expert in identifying the stages of development of larvae or maggots in the body after death. The maggots here had developed from the eggs of a blue or greenbottle fly (known scientifically as *Calliphora erythrocephalus*). Flies' eggs are usually laid in daylight and in warm weather hatch on the same day. The first development of the maggot occurs after 8–14 hours, the second after 2–3 days and the third, the generally recognized fully grown or developed maggot familiar to fishermen, after some 5–6 days, before the maggot develops a shell or pupa. Allowing time for the flies to reach the body, some 11–12 days could have elapsed since Thomas's death allegedly on 16–17 June).

The trial, particularly regarding the role of the entomologist, Professor McKenny-Hughes, was not without incident. I attended court daily, sitting behind Quintin Hogg, who conducted proceedings in a manner entirely dissimilar to that of Ralph Cusack, the prosecuting counsel. Hogg had case papers strewn far and wide, not only on the lectern provided for that purpose but also over the broad curved wooden bench in the Council Chamber being used at Gloucester Assizes. By contrast, Crown counsel was a model of precision, all papers neatly confined to his lectern. Indeed, at one point Cusack remarked to Hogg about his proclivity for entering Cusack's space, so to speak, adding jocularly that it seemed Hogg required sight of papers other than his own bundle.

Giving evidence, ahead of the entomologist's appearance, I was asked my qualifications and experience, the former including my Diploma in Medical Jurisprudence from the

Apothecaries of London. I was surprised to be asked by Cusack, no doubt prompted by Simpson, if it was correct that, when I'd sat for the examination, the senior examiner had been none other than Professor Keith Simpson! The jury saw the amusing side of this forensic entanglement.

Hogg had a difficult time extracting any meaningful information from the entomologist, McKenny-Hughes, who described the proclivities of maggots. Flies, he said, were not, as suggested by Mr Hogg, liable to lay their eggs at midnight. No bluebottle fly laid eggs other than during daylight hours. The entomologist became increasingly involved in the academic side of fly or maggot infestation, so much so that Hogg realized he was getting precious little practical and relevant information from him on the matter, much to the amusement of the court and the frustration of Hogg. Brittle was found guilty of what the judge described as a brutal murder and sentenced to life imprisonment.

Simpson refers in his book to the expectation of a vigorous cross-examination, but I realized that the only medical defence available concerned questions of the possibility of the injury to the voicebox occurring post-mortem, which I had discarded as being tendentious.

Simpson, I thought, exaggerated when he referred to the decisive nature of the maggot evidence, as the case was considered in its entirety by the jury as they came to their firm decision of guilt – unlike the DPP, who had been less than assertive months earlier when formulating a charge of murder. Simpson stated that the stage of development of the maggots indicated a time interval of 11–12 days. If the deceased's body had been taken from Gloucester to Bracknell immediately after death occurred, he was correct in inferring that a time longer than twelve days could have resulted in the maggots forming pupae. It might have been better to allow a time interval of 8–12 days within which the deceased met his death, taking into account the weather conditions – warm summer – when fly eggs could develop earlier and more quickly. This would have covered the time when the three witnesses said they saw the deceased alive.

Occasionally a case arises where there is a conflict of opinion as to whether a death is due to natural causes or to some external agent. An industrial case in which I was involved concerned a worker in a factory who was repairing a broken electric lathe when he collapsed and died. At the subsequent inquest the cause of death was given as an unusual condition, hydrocephalus, which causes swelling and enlargement of the cavities within the brain without impairing intellect or memory. The effects on the brain vary from minor to severe. 'Water on the brain' is an accurate translation of the technical name 'hydrocephalus'. The dead man had been using an electrical tool to repair a defect in the revolving belt.

At the inquest the coroner drew the attention of the jury to possible verdicts: if electricity had played a part, it was an accidental death; it could have been a result of natural causes, due to unexpected effects of hydrocephalus; if they were unsure of the circumstances surrounding the cause of death, an open verdict could be returned. The verdict they gave was one of accidental death, but the cause of death given by the coroner for the death certificate was hydrocephalus. Obviously these statements were contradictory.

Subsequently the man's dependants sued the firm on the grounds that electrocution could have been the cause of death. The inquest had heard evidence of four flaws in the electrical circuit involved in the apparatus, and that if a loose wire had touched the casing of the machine it would have become a conductor of electricity. The action for damages involved the views of several experts, including a specialist on hydrocephalus, a neurosurgeon and two forensic pathologists, of whom I was one. Apart from my colleague, Dr Rufus

Crompton, the experts all gave reasons why hydrocephalus was responsible for the man's collapse and death.

Crompton, a neuropathologist as well as a forensic pathologist, was the only one who agreed with my view that electrocution can occur if there is moist contact due to sweat between a defective electrical apparatus and a person's hand. Further, with a wide area of contact there might not be an electrical mark. The man had apparently collapsed quite slowly when engaged on the repair.

The company agreed to a very substantial settlement being made out of court. A letter from the plaintiff's solicitor said that the widow was grateful for the assistance her case had received, the result of which had made a great financial difference between the dependants' penury and her being able to provide for herself and her children.

So it is not sufficient to conclude that a longstanding condition, whatever its nature, was the cause of a death if in fact some other significant condition was present. Some experts cannot see the wood for the trees.

A second opinion is often sought in cases of manual or ligature strangulation, even if the findings are not exceptional. Such was the case when a young boy was found dead at a seaside town in Essex. Examination showed minimal bruising of the neck tissues externally but definite bruising of the upper margin of the voicebox on one side and bruising of the tissues on the other side, in keeping with manual strangulation. There were characteristic asphyxial changes in the tissues.

Francis Camps, the pathologist, gave a firm opinion that the pressure on the neck had been exerted for thirty seconds, as he thought it would take thirty seconds to show asphyxial changes – not necessarily severe pressure, as he put it, but possibly maintained after the child had died. His view was based on an article written by Camps himself in 1959; I myself thought it impossible to define a time during which pressure must be applied under such circumstances to produce asphyxial changes.

Often the assailant may, perhaps because of his emotional state, have no idea of the time interval; for example, examination of the victims of Dennis Nilsen, the serial killer, confirmed that the time Nilsen maintained pressure on the neck before the victim's sudden collapse varied widely, even in instances when the victim recovered. It is also well known that persons who have survived strangulation can show most marked asphyxial changes. Unfortunately, forensic medicine is a subject which does not encourage objectivity, and statements as to asphyxia, for instance, are purely speculative. Similarly, it is extremely difficult to ascertain the timing of superficial injuries, particularly bruises.

An amusing and surprising case I encountered was a death which was investigated by my late friend Professor Hugh Johnson. I had known Hugh since the time he had joined Francis Camps at the London Medical School Forensic Department. After many years of being second-in-command to Camps, he had somehow found himself left a little behind and out in the cold in the Camps entourage, but was fortunate to be able to start a subdepartment at St Thomas's Hospital, where he dealt with many well known murder inquiries.

The case was that of an elderly white man who had been involved in a minor assault with a coloured man. It was alleged that white people on the estate where the two lived had been the target of unpleasant remarks by coloured residents, and the would-be assailant had approached the elderly man to remonstrate with him. A number of blows were exchanged. The white man was punched four or five times quite lightly, chiefly to the ribs. After the attack I understood that the victim had walked downstairs, entered the van brought by police to take him to the station for a statement, and only thereafter collapsed, some 10-15 minutes later.

The autopsy indicated a few bruises on the face and a small one on the left lower chest, but with the fracture of four ribs on the left side of the chest. There was very serious heart disease, with an enlarged heart and scarring of the muscle caused by previous arterial blockage. Johnson gave the cause of death as natural, due to the heart disease; curiously enough, he did not include the fracture as a contributory cause of death, which might have leant weight to the prosecution case. In the lower court he amplified the opinion in his report by stating that emotion and exertion concerned with the fight were likely contributing factors in precipitating death.

My report pointed out that the effect of the fight was the last straw to a man with severe heart disease, and supported it with an article that Donald Teare and I had written on the medico-legal aspects of heart disease which referred to this sort of event. John Mortimer QC took the case for the defence – it was maybe one of his last trials before he abandoned an active practice in chambers. His down-to-earth manner brought a breath of fresh air to the stuffy courtroom. Mortimer unexpectedly unearthed pithy facts that nobody had considered. After he had questioned numerous witnesses, it was obvious that a much longer time than anybody had realized had passed before the deceased's collapse. His trenchant views had a blistering effect on the pros-ecution case, which was dismissed.

It was a forensic tour de force, piecing together information available from witnesses to pinpoint the time between the inci-dent and the collapse of the victim. I was not aware of this lapse of time, as in order to be so I would have had to have read all the witnesses' statements, which in fact I had not been given. I can only presume that the police had not knitted together the time sequence, and that nor did Johnson know about the matter.

Most defence experts merely confirm the findings of the initial pathologist. What usually matter are differences of opinion, or shades of differences, that come to light, as in one case concern-ing a woman who was found lying face-downwards on the floor at home with scissors in her chest. One blade had entered the middle of her upper chest, passing through the very substantial breastbone to enter the heart sac and cause a fatal haemorrhage.

The husband was accused of stabbing his wife, who had consumed quantities of gin and wine on the day the incident took place. She had apparently tried to slash her wrist a few weeks before while in an hysterical condition. With five to six feet between them, the husband had picked up the scissors and thrown them. They stuck in her chest and she fell to the floor. Donald Teare carried out the autopsy, and there was nothing to criticize in his findings.

Solicitors for the husband wanted to know whether it was possible for the chest wound to have been self-inflicted, particularly in view of the woman's history. Such wounds are extremely rare in women (although I did come across an example some years later, where the wound was thought originally to be the result of a homicidal attack). I believed it highly unlikely that the woman herself could have driven the scissors through the dense sternum or breastbone, and neither did I agree with the view that the scissors could have done this if thrown in the manner described.

It transpired that the accused had trained in martial arts, and was probably capable of throwing an object such as a pair of scissors with greater force and skill than normal. He had stated that at the time he threw the scissors his arm had been outstretched, so that his hand at the moment he released the scissors might have been only three feet or so from his wife's chest as she rushed towards him. I should have paid more attention to this additional information and concluded that such a scenario was possible, even if still unlikely. I was not in the event called to give evidence; I had suggested that, because of my views on the matter, the defence solicitor would be better off employing another pathologist.

The following year I received a nice letter from the firm,

stating that their client had been found not guilty of murder; instead he had been declared guilty of manslaughter and sentenced to just one day's imprisonment. An experiment had been carried out in court to show that thrown a pair of scissors could strike a target with more force and penetration than could be achieved through a simple stabbing motion.

Battered babies are all too common nowadays but it took many years before doctors, pathologists, police and the judiciary recognized the seriousness of such cases. In 1946 Dr Caffey, an American radiologist, noticed that some young children attending his department showed both multiple fractures and head injuries but it took another ten years before the findings were recognized as being due to wilful injuries. In England Francis Camps, in his book on Forensic Pathology in 1956, made no allusion to the condition. Even nowadays, the concept of shaking baby injury is debatable. The hallmark of these injuries is that they occur when one or other parent is present. They are then explained away by falls or unusual impacts and that provided the child recovers, they clear up. Such injuries caused maliciously must have been occurring in the community for many years but had been accepted as part and parcel of the trauma of growing children. In this country in the 1960s medical witnesses found their testimony difficult to be accepted in Court. On one occasion I found myself being mildly reprimanded by a judge as to the explanation of a ruptured liver in an infant being caused by direct violence, rather than a simple fall. A case that brought the matter to the forefront was that of R. v. Dean in 1965 when Michael Dean was charged with murdering his two babies and sentenced to death. This was at a time when the Bill to end hanging was being considered in Parliament. Under the Homicide Act, 1957 two murders became a capital offence when committed at different times. Dean was found guilty but later reprieved by the Home Secretary.

In December 1963, a four-month-old girl was found dead in

her cot. As the doctor, called by her father, noticed bruising on her body, he reported the matter to the Coroner. The local hospital pathologist, Dr Henderson, a man of considerable experience, carried out an autopsy in the presence of two police officers and found some serious internal injuries – an extensive fracture of the skull requiring considerable force for its infliction and also a rupture through the substance of the liver with haemorrhage. At the request of the Coroner, Professor Francis Camps took over the case, reviewed it and it became the subject of an inquest where an open verdict was returned. Later, in October 1964, after Dean had married Susan Moor, the mother of the previous victim, their five-week-old baby was found dead. His father had picked him up from his cot after feeding him and carried him downstairs. Professor Simpson examined the body and found numerous bruises scattered principally on the abdominal wall and, internally, a ruptured liver which his father attempted to explain by a fall the baby sustained against his knee when he picked him up from his cot. Following the second death, Dean was arraigned on a count of causing both deaths and was convicted at the Old Bailey. When asked by the solicitors acting on behalf of Michael Dean to carry out a second autopsy on the second victim and review both cases, I could only agree with the straightforward unexceptional findings. It was a tragedy no further action was taken following the death of the first child.

Since the case of Helen Smith in 1979, coroners have been obliged to hold an inquest when a body is returned to this country following a death that is unnatural. Smith, an English nurse, allegedly met her death following a fall in Jeddah, Saudi Arabia. Her father led a long campaign to apportion blame on account of his view that her death was a murder. (In fact, as far as I know, her body still awaits burial in a Leeds mortuary.)

Autopsies abroad vary greatly in standard and extent, according to the particular country's medico-legal system. It is not unknown for sealed coffins to return to this country containing the body of the deceased from which the internal organs have been removed and replaced by sawdust. Not a pleasant thought. To some extent, the pathologist and coroner have to rely on the history and case details. On other occasions a partial autopsy may have been carried out but vital organs not examined; sometimes organs are removed and not returned; exceptionally, an external autopsy incision may have been made but nothing further. In accidental deaths, it is important that tests for toxicology are done, but they seldom have been. The best one can hope to be sure of is that the body is well preserved.

The well known actor Roy Kinnear died in Spain in September 1988. He had fallen from a horse while galloping over a bridge with Michael York, Oliver Reed and Frank Finlay during the shooting of the film *The Return of the Musketeers*, and had died some 24 hours afterwards in a Madrid hospital, the cause of death being given as heart failure brought on by traumatic shock. Kinnear, aged 54, had been treated in three different Spanish hospitals after the fall – the hospital local to the incident in Toledo, another hospital, and subsequently the clinic in Madrid. His widow, Carmel Kinnear, and Dr John Gayner, medical adviser to the principal insurers of the film industry, pressed for a second post-mortem and inquest into the circumstances of the case.

Kinnear was of shortish stature but rotund; he was clearly heavily built, and the fall was said to have caused a fracture of the main joint of the pelvis in the lower abdomen, which had in turn caused profuse internal haemorrhage and circulatory failure. Although it had been vital in order to keep him alive that a reasonable blood pressure be maintained, there was evidence that proper fluid-balance charts had not been made; this negligence might have affected his kidneys.

His body was flown back to this country and came into the jurisdiction of Dr John Burton, HM Coroner for the outer district of west London. I carried out the examination. There proved to be two fractures of the pelvis, one in front and one on the left side at the back of the hip girdle. The fractures I found and the haemorrhage that had subsequently occurred had caused his death. There was no evidence of heart disease either causing or contributing to the death. The fractures could have been immobilized and the significant haemorrhage and shock subsequently reduced, but this would have required intensive treatment – close monitoring of pulse and blood pressure, and the replacement of body fluid by extensive blood transfusions.

I received appropriate notice to make time available to attend proceedings at the Royal Courts of Justice in the Strand, and the case was in due course settled, with substantial damages being awarded to the widow. Perhaps the outcome would have been different if the accident had occurred in this country, where treatment in an intensive-care unit could well have been successful.

One quasi-forensic case – certainly a medico-legal one – which gave me considerable satisfaction when it was successfully completed concerned a long and hard battle on behalf of a war widow. The British Legion and, in particular, Councillor Richard Goodridge, Sheriff of Carmarthenshire, took up the widow's case claiming a pension due to the death of her husband while a serving soldier in 1941. David Davies, a grocer's assistant aged 33, lived with his wife in Kenfig Hill in South Wales. They had been married for some three months when he enlisted in the Army in December 1940. According to his records he was, on examination for enlistment, passed A1. He joined a unit of the Royal Artillery. He had had no previous known serious illnesses. He came home on leave in February 1941, and just four days later he collapsed while visiting his old place of employment. He was taken home, where his general practitioner certified death.

It may seem quite extraordinary nowadays, but this same GP

also carried out, at the request of the coroner, a post-mortem examination – not only did he carry out that procedure, but he did so in the front room of the deceased's house! This piece of information came to light when Councillor Goodridge met a neighbour of the deceased who had lived next door, in the same house, for fifty-five years. The neighbour remembered the incident well.

In those days it was not particularly unknown for GPs to carry out post-mortems on behalf of the coroner, and in some areas it was quite commonplace, owing to the lack of pathologists; indeed, I can remember my father as a general practitioner carrying out a post-mortem, albeit in a proper mortuary with facilities. It is almost beyond belief, however, that such an examination was conducted in the home of the deceased. One wonders how the widow and the relatives must have felt.

The post-mortem revealed that there were several vegetations, rather like minute fragments of seaweed, on the valves of the deceased's heart, and the GP-cum-pathologist thought it was a sign of rheumatic heart disease. He gave the cause of death rather vaguely as 'dissociation of the ventricles', which means very little except to indicate that the heart had failed.

In 1941 the widow appealed for a pension on the grounds that her husband's death had been caused or aggravated by his military service, but the plea was rejected. Fifty-four years later, when she was 86 years of age, it was again rejected, as it was considered that his heart condition must have been present before he joined up. The reason for the long period between the two applications was that, after her husband's death, she had remarried. She was now a widow again, and was requesting a pension to cover the time between the death of her first husband and her remarriage and again for the time following the death of her second husband.

In January 1996 Councillor Goodridge approached me for my views. After studying the case, I thought that, had the man had rheumatic heart disease on entering the Army, as was alleged in the post-mortem report, he should have exhibited some signs, such as heart murmur, when he was being clinically examined on enlisting – indeed, that he would have been rejected for service. It was clear that, if he had been suffering prior heart disease, any form of training might have had a deleterious effect on it.

It was only in March the following year, that the Pension Appeals Tribunal decided that Gunner Davies's death due to rheumatic heart disease had been aggravated by service. Naturally, Goodridge and the man's widow were very pleased with the award, particularly coming as it did at the end of an often seemingly hopeless legal battle. The case may seem trivial, unworthy of mention or comment, but it illustrates how unyielding the determination of an individual can be in the pursuit of justice. The precise cause of Gunner Davies's death will never be known, but justice was done at last.

Chapter Six

Men are Stabbed and Women are Strangled

The title of this chapter overstates the truth, of course. A rider is that, not infrequently, the murders of men are associated with alcohol, vendettas and racist attacks while the murders of women are often related to marital arguments or sexual assaults taking a turn for the worse.

Over the past thirty years the distribution of hard drugs in the community has led to many more violent deaths; a case in north London indicated the beginning of a trend.

The case occurred back in the mid-1970s. The headlines of the day referred to 'THE GIRL WHO PEDDLED IN DEATH'. The body of the deceased, a 22-year-old Thai student, Laor Rogenkatanyoo, was found in a railway maintenance hut next to Bounds Green Station and the railway line. She was lying in the corner of the hut on cushions, her head and torso at an angle. July that year had been very hot, and when I attended the scene there were fly eggs around the nose and eyelids. She was fully dressed in a nylon anorak and multi-coloured skirt, with no signs of interference or disturbance of her clothing. It appeared that she had been dead for the best part of two days.

Around her neck was a very tight ligature comprising a pair of tights with two knots at the front. In addition there was a bruise across the lower part of the jaw on the left side – and this may well have indicated the main method of assault: overpowering her by placing a hand across the mouth before a ligature was applied and tightened.

The police were initially puzzled for a motive behind this murder, but it transpired that, before arriving in London the previous year, she had been a smuggler of drugs on the Ho Chi Minh trail, bringing heroin to US troops in Vietnam. She had left her west London flat a couple of days earlier ostensibly to join a student coach trip to Cambridge – so how had she ended up dead in a shed in north London? She must have been keeping an appointment with a 'connection' who regularly met her there for drugs. Further information suggested that her customer had suspected she was passing off soap powder as a drug – certainly a motive for murder.

I heard subsequently that a drug pusher was arrested in central London after making a death threat to another woman drug trafficker. This led to him being charged with the death of the girl in north London, and he was found guilty at the Central Criminal Court. It was, therefore, quite by chance that this drug-culture death was solved.

A forensic pathologist seldom has the opportunity to examine an accused person in a murder case, as this task usually falls to the police surgeon, known nowadays as the forensic medical examiner. The murder discussed below involved me with both parties.

A 19-year-old Indian woman was found lying dead on the carpeted floor of their living room when her husband returned home one afternoon, having left for work at 6 a.m. She was fully dressed and lying on her back, and post-mortem changes suggested she had not been dead for long. There were intense asphyxial changes on the face and marks across the front of the neck indicating the previous application of a tight ligature, but there were no marks on the back of the neck. This was in keeping with a form of strangulation known as garrotting. In this case the material used was a broad band of material, and the attacker had approached his victim from behind.

The flat was modern and well furnished, and there were no significant signs of a struggle – although in any case death by garrotting does not lend itself to a very active defence by the victim, who was in this instance a small, slimly built girl.

The CID investigation led to the arrest of an Asian man, a friend of the deceased. Four days later I was asked to examine him as the police had apparently noticed at that late stage some minor scratch marks on him which were fading fast. I did so. He was a powerfully built young person, with a healed scratch just visible within his left ear and more below the ear on both sides of the neck, and just below the collarbone. He alleged the scratches were due to an improperly held razor. Although they were now largely faded and healing, I thought they were more likely caused during the struggle as his victim vainly attempted to defend herself from his clutches by raising her arms behind her and scratching him with her long varnished nails.

He had visited the deceased earlier that day. It was believed an argument ensued and the girl was strangled, although the material used was never found.

There was no cross-examination about her injuries or those of the boyfriend; his explanation of the scratches was not accepted, and he was found guilty and sentenced to life imprisonment.

The death of an even younger married girl, aged just 17, in north London in 1985 gave rise to a remarkable trial. She was found murdered in a van in north London. Her husband, sixteen years older, had left his van on a grass verge and walked to the nearby police station, where he made a statement concerning his wife, whom he said had collapsed in the van after an argument.

Officers went to the scene and found her sitting in the passenger seat of the car, quite dead.

At post-mortem I found she had died an asphyxial death from pressure on the neck. The medical facts of the case, however, were not so straightforward as first appeared. My findings were unusual in that there were only a few small asphyxial haemorrhages in the corner of the eyelids, and none on the skin elsewhere. There were some on the surfaces of the heart and lungs, but these are generally reckoned to be less significant than those found on the outside of the body, particularly above the level of compression on the neck. The brownish-red pressure mark on the neck was also unusual as it was just below the chin on the front of the neck, about one inch long and half an inch wide, while a second irregular mark with abraded edges was just below it and just above the Adam's apple. Moreover, although the subjacent tissues of the neck showed some bruising, there were no fractures of the bones of the voicebox, probably because of her youth.

It was clear that the thumbs of both hands of the accused had been placed securely and very firmly around and across the front of her neck, the fingers extending and encircling her fur-lined coat at the back. His fingers probably gained leverage as they pressed into the back of her seat in the car. This would cause haemorrhage into the deeper tissues and, as the pressure was very firm and sustained, there was little time for surface haemorrhaging into the facial tissues.

I was therefore surprised when the defence submitted that the whole tragic episode had been an accident. The husband, they said, had pulled his van over to the grass verge of the road as they drove home, amid a heated discussion. He brought the vehicle to a halt and leaned over to open the passenger door for his wife to get out, but his arm slipped and his hands went round and/or across his wife's neck. (This defence had not been revealed previously, standard practice in those days.) The defence maintained that it was almost certainly an instance of vagal inhibition when the man's hand made unexpected minor contact with the neck of his wife, who might have been slightly nervous and upset over their disagreement.

After firmly denying the possibility of this scenario, I emphasized that there were minute but definite external haemorrhages with bruising of the neck. The reason there were no massive changes was due to the very firm pressure obliterating the vessels of the neck as they were compressed.

My evidence was heard in court in the presence of an acolyte of Professor Francis Camps, who was advising the defence on the medical evidence. Camps was well known to specialize in unusual and sometimes specious defence submissions, and this was an example. In court, his junior colleague shook his head quite obviously at my utterances – presumably for the benefit of the jury. His histrionics were to no avail. The accused was found guilty.

One can better appreciate the unusual background of this case when one learns that, as became known at the end of the trial, the accused had only three years previously been found guilty of battering his first wife to death. Surprisingly, on that occasion he had been given a conditional discharge by the eminent judge and advocate, now deceased, Mr Justice Scarman. Scarman said in court: 'Please respond to the trust I have put in you and see you bring up your children to be decent and respectable citizens. This is one of those rare cases in which society would be better served in giving your family the advantage of your presence, rather than sending you to prison.' The husband had five children to look after, so there was genuine sense in the learned judge's mind. It also transpired that another man had been paying his wife and the children far more attention than was necessary, which was ostensibly the motive for her murder. The question of diminished responsibility was established in the case, and this enabled the charge of murder to be dealt with in the manner described.

No such plea could be put forward in the matter of his second wife's death, and, indeed, doctors found the accused to be mentally entirely normal. The second marriage had lasted only some six months before coming to this abrupt end. The case for the accused had been very ably presented by Mr Peter Pain QC and, in a plea for mitigating circumstances, he emphasized the need for the man to have access to and care of his large family. To emphasize the accused's resolve, Pain ascertained from him that he had no intention of marrying for a third time. Although the accused was found guilty and given a life sentence, the judge gave him an indeterminate sentence on grounds of manslaughter so that the Home Office would have an opportunity to release him when they were satisfied that the time was right.

There is a wide spectrum of findings in asphyxial deaths, depending on the circumstances of the case and on post-mortem changes; if these latter have developed sufficiently, the passage of time may have obliterated asphyxial changes. Such was the unsatisfactory case, so far as the medical findings were concerned, when I was called to a house in north London where a young couple had rented a room. As they had not been seen for a couple of days and the landlord had previously heard an altercation, the police were called. It was several days after her death that the girl's body was found there, her boyfriend having disappeared. Two days later he turned up at a police station saying he had strangled his girlfriend.

Although decomposition was not advanced, it had obliterated any significant external changes that might have indicated the cause of death. There was just a faded graze over one eyelid and a small bruise on the nose – no asphyxial changes or marks on the neck. The medical cause of death seemed unascertainable until the boyfriend unfolded a story of increasing tension. She had tried to hit him once with a frying pan. He punched her and pushed her away as she approached him again, her arms above her head wielding the frying pan, her neck extended. His hands went round her somewhat long neck and at this point, he said, she collapsed. 'Died of fright' would be a lay term for the event, but medically the only explanation was vagal inhibition, where contact with the sensitive neck skin causes a reflex cardiac arrest. I had no evidence to show strangulation as the cause of death and, other causes being excluded, there was insufficient evidence for the court to continue with a charge of murder.

There was no such difficulty in assessing the medical findings about a 20-year-old Irish girl found dead in a flat in a large Victorian house in Hammersmith, west London, in the summer of 1970, but there were nevertheless a number of problems to be solved.

The young girl, a known prostitute, lived at a house in Talgarth Road, Hammersmith, a short distance from the Broadway. The long road, forming a thoroughfare out of west London, was at that time a street where the houses were in a generally poor state of maintenance. The flat consisted of a bathroom, a kitchen and a small bedroom beyond it. The main room was a bedsitter, the contents of which left one in no doubt that it was used, as described in court, for immoral purposes – in this case prostitution. The principal feature was a double bed with two worn mattresses and a third mattress on top. It was under this composite bed, according to the accused person charged with her death, that he had found her just after midnight on 1 August. He lost little time in informing police of the matter – a good example of the criminal returning to the scene of the crime.

The girl lay on her front with her feet underneath the edge of the bed, a plastic drinks bar on the other side of the bed, and a wig by her arm; there was also a urinary bottle on a small trolley. Numerous photos of girls in suggestive postures and a printed notice with the large letters 'SMILE' were on the mantelpiece.

She was wearing transparent black knickers, a brassiere and a short negligee. There were some superficial marks on the chest, and a prominent ligature mark across the front of the neck: it had the form of a deep brownish-red discoloration, with a smooth outline and sharp margin, running across the side of the neck to fade away on the back of the neck, the characteristic appearance of a person who has been approached and attacked from behind – garrotted, in other words. The mark around the neck was in keeping with having been caused by a strip of pliable plastic which was missing from the side of a television set in the corner of the room.

The cause of death and the circumstances were becoming clear. But how did it all fit in with the story of the victim being found under the bed? The marks on the body showed that she had lain for some hours after her death on her back, as blood had gravitated to the tissues on the back of the body. She must have been subsequently moved and placed on her front, presumably when she was put under the bed for a relatively short time, as a pool of dried secretions from the victim's mouth could be clearly seen on the floorboards near the wall. This opinion was reinforced by the fact that there was a distinct pallid inert-pressure mark on the back of the body. This mark coincided with pressure on her back from one of the supports across the base of the mattress.

A young police officer was designated to be a dummy, and he gallantly lay under the bed for a hour or so to indicate how the pressure mark would develop in that area, although it produced a more livid weal on his back. Whether he was commended by his superior officer I know not, but he deserved to be!

The only matter to clear up was how long she had been dead. She had last been seen at 9 a.m. the previous day. The temperature of the body indicated she had died sometime before early evening, and been left on the floor on her back. Her assailant must have returned, turned her body over, placed it under the bed and, an hour or so later, gone to the police with the story that he had found her there and pulled her out. There was, despite his claim, sufficient evidence to charge him with murder, and he was found guilty at the Central Criminal Court and sentenced to life imprisonment.

Most fatal stab wounds occur as the result of an assault, fracas or fight involving men, and it would be invidious to choose any group as meriting special attention.

Because of its nature and circumstances, together with the considerable press interest it aroused, one case comes immediately to mind. In November 1978 I joined a number of senior detectives – two detective superintendents (one being a chief superintendent) and two detective inspectors (unlike nowadays, when more junior officers would be present at the autopsy) – to investigate a multiple stabbing. It involved the death of John Darke, aged 32, who had at the time of death been involved in the stabbing of a television and film actor, John Bindon, aged 35.

The post-mortem examination took some time as there were nine wounds, one on the back of the body, one on the left leg and the other seven on the chest. The fatal one passed through the substance of the breastbone, a solid structure, and pierced the heart, resulting in fatal haemorrhage. The wound had to have been inflicted with considerable force. Later I examined a sheath knife some six inches long with an inch-wide blade which I thought consistent with the fatal wound. Also retrieved was the knife's sheath, which was inscribed with the name of the girlfriend of the man to be accused, John Bindon.

The stabbing occurred at the Ranelagh Yacht Club in Fulham, west London; despite its name, this was little more than a drinking den, and later it burnt down. The prosecution alleged that Bindon had accepted a £10,000 contract to kill Darke, but in court Bindon maintained that Darke had attacked him with a knife saying, 'This is for you, Bindon, you gonna go'; thereupon

Darke had stabbed him in the chest and also cut him across the throat. Following this there was a general free-for-all involving other men, who were later accused of causing an affray. Darke received stab wounds from which he died.

In spite of his serious injuries, Bindon, with the help of his girlfriend, was able to make his way to Dublin where, from a hospital bed, he contacted police. He admitted stabbing Darke in self-defence, and subsequently at the Central Criminal Court was found not guilty of murder, the judge in his summing up mentioning extensive provocation.

Subsequently Bindon said of the deceased man Darke, 'I often look down at the floor and think – is it hot enough for you down there Darkie?' Perhaps the most unlikely feature of the case was that Bindon was able physically to flee the country and find his way to Dublin. Truth is stranger than fiction.

Bindon died in 1993, aged 50, after an extraordinary life as an actor, appearing in films and television series including *The Sweeney* and the private-eye series *Hazell* – an episode of which could almost have been a rehash of the events surrounding Bindon's trial. He was an acquaintance of royalty and had part-nered a number of well known models and actresses. He had grown up in, as he put it, 'the back streets', and had done time in Borstal and prison. He usually played tough-guy roles, and was known as 'Biffo the Bear' to his friends.

Finally, to reverse the thesis of this chapter's title, here is a case where a husband was strangled by his wife – not in a crime passionnel, or in a situation where a raffish excitable woman, leading a Bohemian life, has an opportunity to strangle her faithless lover. The tragedy occurred in an unlikely setting on a council estate north of London, in Hertfordshire.

I was at a forensic meeting in London when I received a call concerning a suspicious death. I was soon on my way to meet Detective Superintendent McGuinness, who was in charge of the case. I arrived at the terraced house on the edge of the estate where, in the front room, I was shown the body of a 33-year-old man lying on the carpeted floor. Apart from his jacket, which lay on a nearby sofa, he was fully clothed, stretched out with his legs slightly apart and his hands and arms by his side. His shirt was unbuttoned at the neck, the collar crumpled and partly covered by a length of tie which crossed over the front of his chest. There was a long, serrated carving knife in his right hand.

I carefully raised his forearm to test for rigor mortis, so as to confirm whether or not his fingers had been grasping the knife at the time of death. The knife fell gently to the floor, which meant that he could not have been holding it, as the muscles of the hand would have maintained their contraction around it for many hours; it had been placed in his hand after death, and the fingers wrapped around it. The rest of the body was quite stiff.

The phenomenon of rigor mortis is accentuated and accelerated if the victim is in a state of great physical tension and excitement. A bizarre but striking illustration was seen among cavalrymen who had the misfortune to be decapitated by cannonballs during the Charge of the Light Brigade at the Battle of Balaclava. They remained sitting bolt upright in their saddles, frozen, so to speak, in a condition of instantaneous rigor.

Here in Hertfordshire there were more mundane matters to consider, in particular relating to the knife.

The other occupant of the house at the time of the death, apart from a small child asleep upstairs, had been the wife, who said she had been attacked by her husband wielding a carving knife when he returned home after midnight the previous evening. 'I was frightened – grabbed his tie, pulled it tight and kept on pulling it. We both fell to the ground. He stayed there, not moving. The knife in his hand had fallen out on to the floor, so I picked it up, put it in his hand, then took it out, wiped it on my dressing gown and finally replaced it as it had been when he tried to attack me.'

At the autopsy I found there were intense congestion and asphyxial changes in his face and the characteristic deep indentation of a ligature across the front of his neck, with some scuffing of the skin around – suggesting that he had possibly tried in vain to release the pressure of the tie, dropping the knife accordingly. The deeper tissues of the neck were suffused and bruised, and there was a fracture of the cartilage of the voicebox, all signs of sustained pressure over some time, with the tie pulled tightly across his neck.

According to the wife, a short slender person, he had returned home the worse for drink, a not infrequent occurrence. A neighbour had heard ranting and raving in the road outside. Once inside his house, he looked out of the window, said he was going to kill the boy next door, and then reappeared from the kitchen with the knife, saying to his wife, 'Right, you're next.'

Detectives were puzzled by a number of incongruous features. The man's jacket lay on the settee and his head was next to the settee's front, as if he had slipped or possibly been pulled to the floor from this settee. Some pink talcum-like powder was strewn around his body and on the face and clothing, and the fire irons were scattered at random on the carpet. There were three long slashes on the back of the armchair nearby.

Initially it was considered a possibility that the accused might have taken the opportunity to deal, once and for all, with her unpleasant and drunken husband as he lay in a stuporous state on the sofa, seizing his tie, dragging him to the floor and arranging a scene of disturbance. According to this scenario, she used her powder-compact mirror pressed against his mouth to check in case he was still breathing, then put the knife into his hand. Such would have been the stuff of Agatha Christie but, as later became apparent, this reconstruction was invalid.

The wife was charged and her trial took place several months later in the crown court.

The court was full, and the defendant appeared very nervous, whispering her plea of Not Guilty. In his opening speech her defence counsel read her account and affirmed that she was ready to give evidence if necessary. I was then called to give my evidence relating to strangulation as the cause of the man's death, and opined that the tie had been pulled across his neck forcibly and with sustained pressure. I had also found that the deceased's alcohol level was high enough to indicate a state of advanced intoxication. The accused's counsel gave a vigorous plea that she had at all times acted entirely and wholly in self-defence, and maintained that there was therefore no case for her to answer. Additionally, there was nothing to show intent, which would necessarily be the core of any successful murder charge. After an interval during which legal points were submitted, the judge said that he agreed entirely with the facts of the case and also with defence counsel's submission, so on the second day of the trial he stopped the case. The jury acquitted the defendant, and she was able to leave the court to be reunited with her friends and family.

Chapter Seven

The London Nude Murders

Cause célèbre murders attract massive interest from media and public alike, and the deaths of six prostitutes in west London between January 1964 and January 1965 offered no exception. The murders were all committed in a similar way and had unusual features.

It was a cold February morning in 1965, the 16th of the month, when I was called to examine the last of these bodies, that of a naked woman, found earlier that day by a man who worked at a factory on the nearby trading estate. At first sight he thought the corpse was a tailor's dummy, as it was virtually completely hidden from view, lying close to the wall of a brick shed – an extension of the factory building – on a very narrow grass verge, with a fenced railway embankment on the other side.

It took me only a short time to motor from St George's Hospital, Hyde Park Corner, to the site at Acton where I met Detective Superintendent Baldock and Detective Inspector Crabbe, who were in charge of the investigation. They showed me the body as it had been found, lying on its back, almost concealed by grass and thistles. It had all the appearances of being well preserved, with some generalized pallor but no obvious injuries. There was slight sogginess of the skin of the back, suggesting that it had lain where it was found for a short period of time.

The woman was identified as Bridget (Bridie) O'Hara, a slimly built person of, I gathered, similar height to the previous five victims. Subsequent examination showed no sign of strangulation and, apart from a few possible abrasions or areas of pressure on the skin on the right side of the neck, the body was remarkably free of interference. Small haemorrhages were present in the face and eyelids, indicative of an asphyxial form of death, as had been noted on the previous victims. Her dentition was poor, and the upper incisor teeth were missing. There was no obstruction of the air passages. Perhaps the most important finding was that, although she was naked, the clear imprints of her brassiere and panties or knickers were evident on her back. Although the outer clothing was nowhere to be seen, it was clear that her underclothing had been left on until removal at least four to six hours after her death. If that removal had been done *in situ*, the person who had dumped her there was familiar enough with the locale to know that the spot where she had been found gave almost complete protection from prying eyes. I gave the cause of death as asphyxia due to pressure on the face.

Some forty specimens were taken for laboratory investigation at Scotland Yard, where forensic scientists identified particles of paint in the debris taken from the skin surface, corresponding on analysis to the paints and colours used in car workshops for paint-spraying – a finding that subsequently proved to be vital in determining where her body had been lying before being dumped on the verge.

The deceased woman had come to London with her husband a few months before her death. They had separated, but her husband saw her on 11 January, some four weeks before she was found, and others had seen her later that evening leaving a public house at closing time.

It is important to mention the previous victims. The first was

Hannah Tailford, last seen alive on 24 January the previous year, 1964, when she left her home in south London, distinctively dressed for her work in the West End. She had initially arrived in London from the north of England. Ten days after her disappearance she was found on the foreshore of the River Thames in west London, naked, with her pants in her mouth. At the time it was thought possible that her death could have resulted from her involvement in blackmailing one or more clients, as she was known to be a participant in unusual sexual practices at parties arranged in houses in Mayfair and Kensington, as well as for entertaining clients and then later compromising them with photographs she had taken. It was just possible she had been drowned by accident, the gag preventing her from crying out, as is sometimes seen. There was at that stage no cast-iron certainty that she had been murdered, and the coroner's inquest returned an open verdict, as the circumstances surrounding her death were not clear.

When the next victim, Irene Lockwood, was found on the foreshore of the Thames some two months later, also naked, perceptions altered. This second death was followed by the arrest of a man who had made a confession to Lockwood's murder, and he certainly appeared to know more about the case than had been revealed in the press. He was sent for trial at the Central Criminal Court, where he soon withdrew his previous statements, saying they had been the result of too much drink, depression, and a wish to draw attention to himself. He was found not guilty after a six-day trial, and discharged.

Some sixteen days later the body of Helen Barthelemy was discovered in a small driveway in Brentford, not far from where the first two bodies had been found. She was naked and, for the first time, marks of missing underclothing were seen on her waist; some front teeth were also missing, although not apparently due to a blow or violence.

By this time – three murders down – the public had become

increasingly aware, interested and concerned, and the police were warning girls operating in west London to be careful.

Three months elapsed before, on 14 July, a fourth body was found. This was Mary Fleming, discovered in a cul de sac in Chiswick, west London, with a denture missing from her mouth. The person who had dumped her body had narrowly escaped detection, as some painters working overnight to redecorate some rooms of an adjacent building had heard a car being reversed and later returning to the area, and also in the cul de sac itself. The bodies of both Barthelemy and Fleming had acquired the same telltale paint particles that would later be found on Bridie O'Hara.

On 2 November a fifth body, that of Margaret McGowan, was found covered by wood and leaf debris in Hornton Street, Kensington, a narrow street running parallel to fashionable Kensington High Street and, curiously enough, not far from Kensington Borough Mortuary. Again she was nude, with no trace of clothing anywhere in the vicinity and some evidence of decomposition. She had last been seen some ten days before. McGowan was also known as Frances Brown, and had given evidence at the trial of the osteopath Stephen Ward, the man at the centre of the Profumo Scandal the previous year. Ward committed suicide on the last day of his trial at the Old Bailey. (No connection was ever found between McGowan's death and anyone involved in the Ward case.)

Donald Teare had carried out the examination in the first five cases, and had established that the cause of death was some form of suffocation. The police investigation was in the able hands of the most experienced CID officers in London. In addition, Detective Superintendent John du Rose, later a Deputy Assistant Commissioner of Scotland Yard, took overall charge, masterminding plans and resources in the attempt to solve the murders.

The victims were all known for their deviant sexual proclivities. They were all between 5ft and 5ft 2in in height, and solicited their clients among late-night kerb crawlers in west London. All frequented all-night cafes and clubs in the area, and all were dumped near a particular area of the River Thames. In retrospect, their deaths were all attributed to forcible suffocation during violent oral sex.

Du Rose coined the nickname Jack the Stripper to account for the activity of their predator, the title harking back to the infamous Jack the Ripper, who murdered at least five prostitutes in the East End of London in the 1880s. With one exception, the Ripper's victims were viciously murdered and mutilated in dark alleyways. The person responsible was never identified, despite sending notes baiting the police with details of his activities. Over the years at least a hundred books have been written about the case, the authors putting forward different suspects, usually well known personalities from the top echelons of society, whom they think were responsible. Any large bookshop is likely to have three or four Jack the Ripper books on the shelves.

Du Rose flooded the streets of west London with policewomen disguised as prostitutes – a hazardous duty – with a view to finding the killer, and a large number of police officers were deployed to make extensive house-to-house inquiries concerning occupants and, where appropriate, their cars. The CID component grew to some 200 officers and, as the investigation reached its farthest point west, they uncovered the site of the paint-spraying activities.

It was on the factory site next to where O'Hara's body had been found. The bodies of O'Hara and some of the other victims had probably been hidden near a transformer at the back of the factory, and the paint spray contaminated their skin with particles. At the inquest in February 1966 where I gave evidence, it was revealed that some 120,000 persons had eventually been interviewed, and 4,000 statements had been taken. The suspects traced as the result of this huge investigation were whittled down to three men. As the net was closing in on one man in particular, evidence of paint flakes having been found in his car and garage, he disappeared.

The murders ceased, and du Rose's view was that the murderer had committed suicide. It was also rumoured that he had been admitted to a mental hospital. However, no arrest was made and no trial or conviction took place. We must bear in mind that, without such events, the man must be considered innocent. As his family and relatives were still alive, the police wished to spare them the full story; they had no knowledge of his activities outside a normal family suburban background. A psychiatrist commenting on the matter said he thought the man responsible for the murders was emotionally crippled in his early childhood, and had had to repress for most of his life his strong subconscious fears, hatreds and sadistic urges. The final words from the police were that the file remained open.

Had these events occurred nowadays, the terms 'serial murders' and 'serial killer' would have been bandied about, but they were unheard-of in the 1960s. For my part, no further court appearance was necessary, of course, but I was to encounter another set of serial murders some eighteen years later, in the case of Dennis Nilsen.

Chapter Eight

Bombs and Bullets

The protracted bombing campaign of the IRA on the mainland of Great Britain between 1970 and 1990 resulted in a number of incidents and explosions which caused considerable damage and many deaths of innocent people. Notable in London were the explosions at the Old Bailey and in Whitehall, and both shootings and bombings in the West End. Working in north London, the City of London and Hammersmith, west London, I was involved in the investigation of several of these crimes – two in 1975, one in 1988 and one in 1992.

On 28 February 1975 it was sheer chance that brought the Provisional IRA to the attention of a plain-clothes police officer who was investigating a series of burglaries in the Hammersmith area. These burglaries had occurred in a street close to Barons Court Underground Station, where a man had been seen acting suspiciously. One of the officers, PC Blackledge, spoke to him. He gave an unsatisfactory answer and ran away. The officer gave chase. Meanwhile off-duty PC Stephen Tibble, aged 21, who had completed his training only a few months previously prior to being posted to nearby Fulham Police Station, was passing by on his motorcycle. (He would normally have been on duty that day, but had exchanged his roster with another officer.) Tibble gave chase as well, overtook the fugitive and dismounted. As the man ran towards him, Tibble spread his arms wide; three shots were fired with a 0.9 mm automatic and the man escaped towards the tube station, subsequently fleeing along the tunnels of the underground railway. PC Tibble was taken to nearby Charing Cross Hospital, where he died some two hours later.

At the post-mortem that I carried out it was necessary to find out what had happened to the three bullets. One had caused a minor injury to the base of Tibble's left hand, and I was told that the bullet had been retrieved from the door of a house near the scene of the incident. The second bullet had passed through the deceased's chest and entered his pelvis, causing a major haemorrhage. The third bullet had followed a rather similar track and involved the main blood vessel of the body, this time causing a fatal haemorrhage. It seemed that Tibble had been in a semi-crouched position when these two bullets struck him.

The search for PC Tibble's killer initially centred on the discovery of a bomb factory in an IRA safe house in a street nearby. A number of IRA sympathizers were arrested, questioned and later released, but further inquiries led to a strong suspicion that the man the police wished to question concerning Tibble's death was a certain William Quinn.

Quinn had a curious and interesting background. He was born in the USA, and grew up in a working-class district of San Francisco. Although his family had no interest in Irish politics, Quinn became increasingly involved and he learned Gaelic. In 1970 he was involved in setting up the San Francisco chapter of NORAID, the organization which raises funds for IRA sympathizers. The following year he volunteered for the Provisional IRA, and he was sent to England three years thereafter.

A year after Tibble's death a warrant was issued for Quinn's arrest on bomb charges, and in 1979, three years later, a murder warrant. He escaped, but was arrested in Eire as a member of the

IRA, and served nine months of a year's sentence in a Dublin prison. The same year he fled back to the USA, where in 1981 he was arrested in his uncle's stationery shop in San Francisco. He would probably have remained a free man but for the increased cooperation between the British and American governments during the period when Thatcher and Reagan were both in power, which had brought about a more sympathetic attitude in the USA towards the British campaign against the IRA. Having been arrested by FBI agents, Quinn spent five years in prison fighting extradition from the USA.

At the time of that arrest he was unaware that he was also being watched by CID officers from Britain. Little did he know that the men who purchased items from his uncle's shop were also securing fingerprints and matching them with those on the wrapper of a mail bomb which had been found some years previously. Indeed, Quinn was believed to have sent bombs to prominent people and to have been involved in the planting of bombs at Aldershot Military Barracks and other places.

In February 1988, thirteen years after Tibble's murder, Quinn was jailed for life following a trial in the Central Criminal Court. He had finally been caught as he boarded a ferry from Ireland.

One of the most disturbing IRA murders in the 1970s was that of Ross McWhirter, on 27 November 1975. McWhirter was a former track athlete, a sports commentator, and the compiler with his brother Norris of *The Guinness Book of Records*. He was sponsor of a reward scheme for the apprehension of those responsible for IRA crimes of violence.

On the night in question McWhirter's wife had been out. She returned home by car just before 7 p.m., when it was already dark. As she backed the car into the garage two men appeared, demanding the car keys. Terrified, she handed these over and then went to the front of the house, where her husband met her at the door. Two shots were fired and Ross McWhirter collapsed. The men got into the car and drove off.

I carried out an examination of McWhirter's body later that same evening. His clothing was heavily bloodstained, and I found a bullet wound, a little under a quarter-inch across, on the right side of the head. The bullet had passed through the skull causing, on the left side, very severe and indeed fatal damage. A second bullet hole ran through the abdominal wall to the pelvis. The assailant had fired two bullets, one non-fatal and then the fatal shot, probably fired as McWhirter turned away after the first.

The two killers proved to be Harry Duggan and Hugh Doherty, the former having pulled the trigger to shoot McWhirter with an Astral Magnum revolver. Subsequently they were arrested and sentenced in 1977 to thirty years' imprisonment, being found guilty of murder and causing explosions.

Before their arrest, however, the two gained notoriety in December 1975 for their part in the gang of four, who held hostage the two occupants, husband and wife, of a flat in Balcombe Street, London. The gang were being chased by police after shooting up Scott's Restaurant, in Mayfair, and invaded the flat as a place to hole up. Six days after the start of the ensuing siege, they gave themselves up. The police were delighted to find the murderers of Ross McWhirter among them.

Ten years passed before I was involved in investigating another IRA crime. On 1 August 1988 Lance-Corporal Michael Robbins, aged 23, was attached to the postal courier division of the Royal Engineers and stationed at Inglis Barracks, Mill Hill, north London. The buildings, established many years ago, occupy a large area. Robbins was in bed that night when an explosion occurred in the accommodation section. The building was demolished, and following the collapse of the building Corporal Robbins was found dead beneath the rubble.

I found he had died not by bomb blast or directly from injuries but from a condition of traumatic asphyxia caused when his chest sustained a pinning injury beneath the rubble. It was thought that the bomb had been planted by the IRA, but no one was arrested and at the inquest the coroner returned a verdict of unlawful killing.

On Friday, 10 April 1992 at about 9.20 p.m. the financial centre of the City of London was rocked by a tremendous explosion which devastated the Baltic Exchange, an important financial centre, and other buildings in St Mary Axe including the Commercial Union Building.

The explosion came from a van parked in the road and packed with some one hundred pounds of Semtex. It was the biggest explosion to that date in mainland Great Britain. On any Friday night in that area the wine bars and restaurants were packed with workers celebrating the end of the week; and on that particular Friday some were additionally celebrating the Conservative victory in the General Election the day before, giving the Tories an unexpected further four years in office.

One witness said there was a noise like thunder, the lights went out and the building in which he was still working – the Commercial Union building – shook as if in an earthquake. A diner in a restaurant only a few doors away from the site of the explosion described a tremendous bang and a blue flash.

The area resembled a battlefield. Nine ambulances came to the scene at the corner of Leadenhall Street and St Mary Axe. Two double-decker buses were requisitioned to take casualties to hospital following emergency calls received by the London Ambulance Service. It was remarkable that only three people were killed.

Those dead were a young man who was a securities dealer, a security guard (found later) and one of four occupants of a car, a 15-year-old girl – the latter a particularly tragic incident. Her father, a chauffeur, had arranged to meet his family outside the

Baltic Exchange, where he was returning his car to the car park. As he did so he saw the car containing his two daughters, a friend and the deceased girl's boyfriend flattened by the explosion, and ran out to find his daughter lying inert on the pavement.

My examination showed the girl must have died instantly due to a piece of metal or a glass shard passing through her head. The second victim, the securities dealer, had sustained a number of injuries to his back, the principal one shattering his pelvis and lower back; there were many metal fragments present, and fatal haemorrhages from blood vessels, probably all caused by flying metal. The third fatality, the security guard, was found the following day lying in the rubble with a number of facial injuries caused by glass and masonry; he had sustained a skull fracture and haemorrhage.

Apart from the human devastation, the damage to buildings was in the order of hundreds of millions of pounds – some estimates said it could even run into the billions.

The City – as in wartime – made a remarkable recovery, and within three or four days most staff had been relocated to other buildings and the financial heart of the City beat again. The IRA subsequently blamed the tragic loss of life on the police not acting promptly on a coded warning, but the police believed the bombers had deliberately misled them as to the location of the bomb.

Subsequently a very stringent system of traffic control was set up. All vehicles and personnel were monitored and the drivers checked as they entered the City boundaries.

Over the years, shooting has increased alarmingly in mainland Britain – as has, of course, crime in general. Clearly the increased availability of guns to the underworld and the relatively detached manner in which these weapons cause death can easily lead to the assailant not being apprehended. Nowadays the tremendous increase in drug-use has led to a matching rise in the gang warfare associated with it, and in the use of firearms to kill drug peddlers who have fallen out of line.

Fatal firearm wounds are sometimes more difficult to interpret than you might think. One has to identify the type of gun and bullet responsible from the markings on the skin surface; follow the track of the bullet internally; work out the distance between the gun and the deceased at the time of the shooting; and, as is always necessary, refer the matter to a ballistics expert, who will give evidence in court.

Occasionally cases of shooting come out of the blue or, in one case, from Africa. This unusual case involved a man who had been working at a telecommunications centre in Zaire. He had been challenged at a checkpoint one night while returning to his base by car, and had allegedly been shot when he stopped.

The body having been brought back to Britain, I found the entrance wound of a bullet in the right arm, and the bullet itself was lodged in the tissues in the base of the wrist, as if he had received the wound while his arm was resting on the open driver's window. The bullet had travelled down the forearm through only superficial tissues. But more sinister findings came to light at the post-mortem I performed on behalf of the coroner. As well as revealing the previous wound, the post-mortem found a series of five stab wounds, two of which, on the man's back, were deep enough to reach the liver. This was quite unexpected. The discovery showed the value of having a post-mortem examination done in this country. The wounds indicated that the man had been hauled out of the car after the shooting and viciously stabbed as he lay on the ground by one or more of the soldiers manning the checkpoint.

At the inquest little further information was available, and the coroner returned a verdict of murder by person or persons unknown. So much for the original story that he had collapsed at the wheel of the car after receiving a warning shot from the guard-post!

A case which also involved stabbing and shooting occurred much nearer home and was of a very different genre, being a crime of passion. There is no English legal equivalent of the continental *crime passionnel*, for which, in recognition of the impassioned state of mind of the killer, sentences are usually relatively lenient. This particular example involved the deaths of a man and woman, whose bodies had, by the time I saw them, been expeditiously moved to a district mortuary after an initial investigation by police officers.

The case was a sad instance of the eternal triangle. Unknown to her husband, a wife had taken a lover. The situation came to light one day when the husband picked up the extension line to make a call and overheard a torrid conversation between the two lovers. Shortly afterwards the 28-year-old woman was collapsing under a welter of stab wounds, twenty-five in all, almost all on the back, with a few on her arms from trying to ward off the blows. The weapon was a five-inch knife, later found. Despite the number of wounds only two reached the inner part of the chest to cause fatal haemorrhage. This hail-storm of wounds would certainly fall into the category of a frenzied attack.

The husband promptly left home and went to the house of the lover, who was sitting enjoying a quiet drink with two friends, his back to the door. Throwing the door open, the husband entered the room and, without more ado, shot the lover in the face as he turned around. The fatal bullet lodged in the victim's spinal column.

At the Central Criminal Court trial the husband was found guilty of manslaughter, and sentenced to nine years in prison. As I write this, some ten years later, he should have finished serving his sentence.

Security guards are always targets for prospective robbers, and there have been many cases of criminals staking out a wages collection with a fatal shooting as a consequence, usually when the robbery goes wrong.

In August 1985 a security guard, Sydney Dundon, preparing to deliver about £16,000 to a dry-cleaning firm in west London was shot in the back by a man with a sawn-off shotgun, who snatched the guard's security bag as he lay dying. Of the four assailants involved, two were never found. However, the man who committed the killing and his getaway driver were soon apprehended. Police found the car half a mile away; the driver's palmprint was on a motorcycle crash helmet inside the car, while the thumbprint of the man who had used the shotgun was found on a cash label belonging to the firm.

The two men, Jerry Alexander and Jonathan Joseph, were charged with murder, and appeared at the Central Criminal Court, where I gave my evidence relating to the post-mortem examination which showed the guard had been shot at close range. There was the characteristic oval entry wound of a single-bore shotgun on the back of the chest, with a few oval pitted marks caused by lead pellets on the skin surface and, internally, a large ragged cavity with damaged ribs and fatal haemorrhaging of the lung and liver, from where many shotgun pellets were retrieved. The paucity of the number of pellets marking the skin surface and the appearance of the entrance wound itself indicated that it had been a close-range shot – fired at a distance of about one foot. Judge Miskin, in his summing up to the jury after the evidence had been heard, said that the guard was a decent hard-working family man, and described the murder as a hideous event.

The man with the shotgun was found guilty and sentenced to seventeen years' imprisonment for manslaughter and robbery. The driver of the getaway car received a lesser sentence, fourteen years.

Another notable security-guard killing was likewise associated with an attempted wages snatch. In June the previous year two Securicor guards were ambushed by two men as they were delivering some £9,000 to an office in Brentford, West Middlesex. Both robbers were armed. One stood outside near a motorcycle at the gateway entrance to the firm's offices, while his accomplice posed as a delivery man waiting by the lift, where he confronted the security guards, demanding the cash. One of the guards managed to throw the cash into the lift and a battle developed between the robbers and the guards. One guard, John McWilliams, a married man of 39, was shot in the chest at close range and fell to the floor, dying; the other was wounded in the leg.

In my examination at Charing Cross Hospital I found that the guard had been hit by two bullets. One had passed through the base of the index finger of the right hand. I found the fatal entry wound just above the right collarbone. The pattern of the skin markings around the entrance hole of the bullet indicated that the shot had been fired at the guard from very close range, almost in contact with the skin. The bullet had passed through the upper chest from the right to the left side of the body, through the lungs, and into the spine, where I found it.

At the scene, crucial evidence against the man who had carried out the shooting, Allan Byrne, lay on the ground – an envelope he had used to hide his revolver revealed his thumbprint. He appeared at the Old Bailey and was jailed for life. His accomplice, Richard Trump, also armed was convicted of murder. Both were also charged with possessing a firearm, attempting robbery, and using a weapon to resist arrest.

As they were convicted, fighting broke out in the public gallery. Relatives of the two men showered leaflets into the court and screamed abuse, claiming there had been a fit-up. Allan Byrne, the man responsible for killing the guard left the dock after the verdict of guilty without waiting to hear his sentence, screaming abuse at the judge. Two years earlier he had been cleared at the Old Bailey on similar charges of armed robbery and shooting a security guard.

Young victims are always the most tragic. Gary Hazell, a young lad only 15 years of age, was found lying on the pavement outside his home in Boreham Wood, Hertfordshire, dying from shotgun wounds and, according to his father, who found him, riddled like a pepper pot. He was dead on arrival at hospital.

It was a strange story. The boy had been killed by a 69-year-old man, who was subsequently charged with murder. There had been an altercation before the fatal shooting when the man had appeared with a shotgun, remonstrating with a group of boys for running through his garden, which they denied. A short time afterwards, when the boys had been playing on the pavement outside his house, one of them was pushed against the gate. The next thing a bang was heard and Gary collapsed.

When I examined him in hospital, I found that the shotgun used had produced a pattern of pellets on his chest which extended across it from the collarbone to the midline, indicating a distance of some twelve yards between the boy and the muzzle of the gun. At the man's trial the defending barrister said that the elderly man was almost blind in one eye and had previously had an operation on the other eye. He had not used the shotgun for years on account of his failing sight, and claimed that at the time of the shooting he had intended to fire the gun into the ground to scare the boys. He pleaded guilty to manslaughter and was given a sentence of just one year in prison.

No other extenuating circumstances were put forward on his behalf, the judge commenting that an act of gross carelessness had led to his appearance in court.

Some years later, I examined a not dissimilar wound on the chest wall which had caused the death of a 17-year-old girl in an accident. In Northwood, Middlesex a group of friends were playing with a shotgun when it inadvertently went off. A close friend of the owner of the shotgun, the girl received part of the discharge of the gun on the right side of her neck and collarbone. She was seen at the Accident and Emergency Department of the local hospital, and was admitted for observation. Having overcome the initial shock and seemingly making good progress, she suddenly collapsed three days later.

I knew that, unless some obvious fatal complication from the firearm wound had occurred, it might be difficult to find the cause of death unless it was something totally unrelated.

Examination revealed small bubbles of air in the main chambers of the heart and in vessels adjacent to its surface. These were not due to any of the post-mortem phenomena which can produce gas formation in the tissues. I thought the distribution of the pellets in the tissues, still clearly visible on X-ray, had led to damage of the main vein to the heart, and that air, which had accumulated in the superficial tissues of the neck following the incident, had found its way into the heart, producing a fatal airlock (or embolism). It was a most unusual occurrence.

Another shotgun death which led to a not guilty verdict at trial led me to Brighton, in Sussex, where I was asked to examine the body of a man who had been taken to the county hospital with a shotgun wound in his upper abdomen. His wife had fired the shotgun about six feet away from him and the pellets had blasted away most of his liver. The report of the police surgeon indicated that the wife herself had well marked areas of injury on her neck, consistent with an attempt at strangulation; there were also a couple of older injuries to her face.

The sitting room in the flat where this had taken place showed some disorder, as you might expect from a struggle, and the gun was found propped up against the wall next to a wardrobe.

The case was heard at Lewes Assizes which, although in the country some miles from London, had become familiar to me from my previous work on the south coast. The wife was accused of the murder of her husband with a 0.4 shotgun. She denied murder, but pleaded guilty to manslaughter. She was fortunate to have the well known advocate Lewis Hawser QC acting on her behalf. He informed the court that, a short time before the husband died in hospital, he had told two nurses that it had all been a terrible accident. The judge said he had no need to call the nurses to give this evidence, and told the wife she should put the tragedy behind her and face the future. He accepted that the incident had been one of unintentional recklessness on her part. A sentence of two years' imprisonment was suspended for three years, so that she left the court a free woman.

Christopher Whittaker was an unfortunate lad – doubly so. First he was unfortunate in the company he kept: petty criminals. Second, his life ended abruptly when he became a victim of those with whom he associated. They had lured him to a graveyard in Willesden, north London – 'they' being a gang of 'back street thieves', as they were later described in court – and murdered him in cold blood with a sawn-off shotgun. The motive was that he had 'grassed' on them to the police. His body was found a little less than a month after the shooting, but it could have remained in its unusual burial place for very much longer if the police had not received a tip-off from a member of the gang, who feared he was next on the list.

Of the three persons accused of murder, the leader was a 32-year-old man, Robert White, who had been, on his own confession, a thief since the age of 9. He had not spent a whole year out of prison since he was 13 years of age. The shotgun responsible for Whittaker's death had been bought for committing a robbery, along with some cartridges, although it was alleged that, to spare the victim, the gang had replaced the lead pellets with table salt – so that he would be hideously wounded but not killed. The gang leader had developed a hatred of 'grassers' during his past prison time, but he had in fact once been a 'grass' himself, while in Parkhurst Prison, and as a result had been forced for his own protection to spend the rest of his sentence in solitary confinement. He assumed (incorrectly) that the 16-year-old Whittaker was a police informer, and that he had been implicated by Whittaker in connection with a stolen car and in an attempted robbery that had been foiled by the police.

The gang decided that the only way to deal with this matter was to dispose of the young boy. He accompanied them to the churchyard on their pretext that they were finding a place to hide stolen goods. As they arrived, there were two blasts from a sawn-off shotgun, and the young boy collapsed. After his death they stripped him of his clothing and took the body a short distance in a car to the vicinity of a sailing club beside a well known lake in north London, the Welsh Harp. With the aid of a pick and shovel they buried him in an allotment at the edge of the lake.

It is not uncommon for murders to be revealed and investigated at weekends, and duly I was called to the scene early one Saturday. England was playing Wales at rugby that day, so I was reluctant to answer the appeal, but I was assured that, as exhumation proceedings were in hand, it was likely we would finish work before the afternoon game.

At the burial site I was struck by the remarkable preservation of the body, no doubt due to its being covered in heavy, wet London clay, which enclosed it and prevented decomposition caused by outside conditions. I confirmed that the victim had been shot twice in the head – once in the face and a second time through the left temple, causing many fractures and brain damage. On X-ray the shotgun pellets could be seen widespread in the tissues. There was no evidence of table salt.

Two of the accused received life sentences and the third member was found not guilty. As the judge commented, this was a brutal murder with a macabre setting in a graveyard, the body being buried where it was unlikely to be found. It was in the first instance police vigilance, noticing the young man's disappearance from his usual haunts, followed by a tip-off that led to the discovery of Whittaker's murder. As the macabre joke had it, this was certainly a grave murder.

A case from many years ago, had it occurred nowadays, might have been described as a contract killing. It could have been the result of some personal vendetta, or it might even just possibly have been a callous way of avoiding paying a taxi fare.

A stationary taxicab had been noticed at the side of a road near a pond in an outer suburb of north London. A passing postman thought he saw the driver slumped behind the wheel and called the police. A short time later I met the detective superintendent in charge and, on opening the near side of the cab, we saw the body of the taxi driver, Ivor Pearce, slumped over the partition between his seat and the luggage compartment. His head rested on the floor, surrounded by a pool of blood. Nearby was an empty cartridge case. It was a cold December day and the deceased was heavily clothed. There was nothing of relevance in his pockets. All that I could tell the police was that he must have been dead overnight and, more significantly, that he had been shot through the back of the head.

The entrance wound was behind his left ear, and the bullet had traversed his head, causing a small exit wound in the left cheek. The wound ran virtually horizontally through his skull. It does not need much imagination to conclude that the taxi driver's passenger must have knocked on the glass partition, as one would do to communicate with the driver, and that, when the taxi driver pulled the glass screen across and inclined his ear to hear the passenger's request, the passenger fired the gun – a small-calibre automatic – from a distance of an inch or so from the victim's head.

Despite very intensive CID investigation, interviewing all the taxi driver's contacts and fares, the police got no further in solving the mystery of the shot taxi driver. Clearly he must have picked up his fare, his killer, the preceding evening, probably late at night, and on the passenger's instruction driven to the rather remote spot where the taxi was found. I can hardly think it was a chance shooting; there must have been a sinister motive. The killer's secret, unfortunately, remains.

Chapter Nine

Unexpected Homicide

When homicide occurs it is usually obvious; it is unusual for it to be discovered by accident, as in two cases from 1967 and 1972.

The first involved a wife and mother, Rose Wilde, in a council house in north London, who had received a head injury and then been strangled without her husband or, for that matter, anyone else who had been in the house except the perpetrator of the crime being aware that there was anything wrong. The deceased woman, aged 62, was found in a small upstairs bedroom, lying on her back on the floor. The local doctor had been called in by the husband when he found his wife, but could give no cause of death, and her body was taken to the mortuary. The matter might have bypassed the coroner's system of investigation into unnatural death had not the mortuary superintendent, John Godsalve, an observant man, noticed some marks on the neck.

There were, indeed, marks on the neck – very distinctive and deep abrasions across the back of the neck, with a wavy irregular pattern, fading away towards the midline on the front. It was an unusual pattern consistent with pressure across the back of the neck and caused by some form of ligature, the appearances suggesting that she could have been dragged along by use of the ligature. There had been nothing to indicate this earlier. The clothing, carefully removed and put aside by the mortuary staff, consisted of a printed pinafore, cardigan, blouse, short-sleeved cardigan, skirt, stockings and the usual under-clothes, all undisturbed.

Asphyxial haemorrhages were present in the eyelids, with bruising between the lip and the gum; the upper denture was present, the lower one missing. More surprising was a depressed fracture of the skull on the left side of the top of the head, a frac-ture that did not extend into the skull base but which was associated with a small area of bruising of the brain on the opposite side. Certainly these injuries could not possibly have resulted from a fall. Indeed, the significance of the depression on her skull became clear when the husband said he had had difficulty in frying an egg, as it kept sliding to the side of the frying pan. Examination of the pan showed a distinct dent in the centre caused by impact with the woman's head, accounting for this phenomenon.

When I was at the house, detectives had outlined chalk marks on the carpet where the deceased was thought to have been lying, and I found a bloodstained denture beneath the dressing-table.

There had been, so it transpired later, considerable disagree-ment between mother and son relating to the latter's forth-coming marriage. No member of the family attended the wedding ceremony.

A few hours before the bridegroom left the home for his marriage, as depicted in a happy wedding photograph, he had, it was alleged, hit his mother over the head with the frying pan, stunning her. Unknown to his father, he had then dragged her up the stairs with a tie, fracturing her voicebox and strangling her, and had left her on the bedroom floor. After the wedding cere-mony he acted as if nothing had happened, and he and his bride travelled to Scotland for their honeymoon. It was there that, two days later, he was arrested and charged with murder.

At his trial at the Old Bailey the son was found guilty of

murder. The judge, Mr Justice Wein, commented that he had never come across such callous conduct.

A similar event in 1972 involved a young woman of 25, Beryl Furzer, a part-time hairdresser who lived in a terrace house on the Great Cambridge Road. A most extraordinary state of affairs led to the discovery of her murder. She was found in the bathroom, dead on the floor. There was a vague history of epilepsy and this, combined with some blood from a cut on the head, led initially to a presumption of natural collapse. The coroner's officer arrived and found more blood than had previously been noted; a doctor came to pronounce death, and mopped up yet more blood. In fact, there seemed no end to the amount of blood on the floor that had been removed by a succession of attendants at the scene. Eventually, blood was even noticed on the ceiling of the downstairs kitchen.

The deceased was taken to the mortuary, where it was noticed that there were a number of cuts on her scalp beneath her long dark hair. When I examined her I found four lacerations on the right side of the head, seven across the top of the head and four on the back of her head, with underlying fractures of the skull and a fatal haemorrhage around the brain. She had been the subject of a frenzied attack with multiple blows from some metal weapon, probably with a rounded end, and the severe head injuries had caused death.

Visiting the house subsequently I saw blood splashes on the wallpaper of the stairs and landing, and on the opposite side above the arch of the stairs.

At first the investigation drew a blank, but it became apparent the deceased was acquainted with a man who lived nearby. He had left the area, but was traced to Dublin, where he was found in possession of a portable radio taken from the dead woman's house. He was found guilty of the charge of murder and sentenced to life imprisonment.

Murder may go undetected, particularly if a plausible

explanation is put forward, or there are no obvious suspicious circumstances.

'Time of death, Doc?' It's a cliché from any of countless television crime series, of course. The television pathologist clad in clothing acquired from a second-hand shop adopting a somewhat patronizing attitude towards the detective colleague who asks the question. It's not quite like that in real life . . .

I am regularly faced with this time-of-death problem, and sometimes establishing an answer can be crucial to the course of an investigation. A striking example concerned the death of a 57-year-old housewife. Her husband was a taxi driver.

On the morning of 1 May 1986 she should have been working as the manageress in her daughter-in-law's shop in north London. She was a person of remarkably regular habits – someone said you could almost set your watch by her. She always phoned her daughter-in-law on arrival at the shop in the morning at 9.30 a.m., but today she did not do so. On phoning the older woman's home, the daughter-in-law obtained no reply. Later, worried by her continued nonappearance at the shop, the daughter-in-law went round to the house. As she approached she noted that the front bedroom window was partially open – quite a normal occurrence – and discovered that the front door was unlocked, which was not so usual: it would normally have been locked if her mother-in-law had been upstairs for any length of time, as for example while dressing or bathing.

When the younger woman went in she noticed the breakfast things on the worktop in the kitchen, the strip light on and likewise the television. The bed upstairs in the room with the open window was unmade. After going through the rooms, she found her mother-in-law lying on the floor of the small rear bedroom, face-down, wearing a long nightdress. She called an ambulance, which arrived promptly. The police were summoned, as an ambulance attendant said she saw a suspicious mark on the dead woman's neck. During the daytime the deceased always wore jewellery, in particular a gold pendant, two heavy gold chains and a thin gold chain around her neck, plus wristlets. Apparently she never took off the chain around her neck, yet it was missing when she was found.

There was no sign of a break-in to the house or any form or suggestion of a struggle, but at the post-mortem later that afternoon I found clear evidence of ligature strangulation, in keeping with the chains on her neck being used for that purpose.

At this point it is interesting to note how extremely regular were the habits of the husband and wife in the early morning. They usually rose about 7 a.m., and the wife would put on her dressing gown, open the window, turn on the television and made a cup of coffee for her husband and a cup of tea for herself, leaving a second tea-bag in the tongs for use later. The latter tea-bag was in evidence on the kitchen worktop, with a half-drunk cup of tea nearby and an empty coffee mug in the sink. It therefore appeared that the couple had had breakfast while, as was their custom, the television was on for the early-morning news. The husband had left the house in his taxi for work at about 7.30 a.m.

On this particular day the husband said he had to phone a client before leaving. While he was doing this, his wife was on her way upstairs, apparently to dress for her own work. He went out without seeing her again. He quietly and firmly denied at all times that he had had anything whatsoever to do with her death.

If the husband had been responsible for strangling her, the time of the killing would be of vital importance. Should it be shown that his wife had died after 7.30 a.m., there was no way he could have been responsible. The scenario in the kitchen – the coffee, tea, television and phone call – would all be important corroborative or circumstantial evidence as to his innocence. On the other hand, the scenario might have been fabricated with exactly that in mind.

Sadly, the initial investigation in the house was somewhat

slipshod. No temperature had been taken at the scene while the body was lying on the floor and the police surgeon who was called did not examine the body other than to certify death.

Luckily I was able to carry out the autopsy within three-quarters of an hour of the body being removed from the house – that is, some five hours after it had been found. This short interval of time was particularly fortunate in relation to the distribution and development of hypostasis, which was clearly visible on the front of the body, although there were far more marks of hypostasis on the back. Hypostasis forms as gravity causes the blood to seep into dependant soft tissues according to the position of the body at the time of death, so the fact that it was present on both sides and far more prominent on the back indicated that some person had, at some time after death, shifted the body from supine to the prone position in which it was finally found.

Post-mortem lividity (hypostasis) takes at least one to two hours to develop and after some four hours, regardless of any movement of the body after death, it remains in its initial distribution, so it was clear that this lady had been dead for about four hours before her body position was changed.

I visited the house subsequently and noticed how warm it was; indeed, the thermostat settings on the boiler were easily available to police. It became known that the husband had often complained that the house was too warm, and had taken to overriding the time clock on occasions, contrary to his wife's wishes.

At my examination at 4 p.m. I found her body temperature to be 83°F; i.e., it had fallen some 15°F since the time of death from the usual 98°F. A body loses heat according to many factors, chiefly the surrounding temperatures but also the build of the deceased person and the clothing. Heat is lost by conduction, convection and, to a minor degree, radiation. Also, of course, the rate of cooling depends in part on currents of air circulating around the body. As a general rule, a body which loses heat slowly to room temperature does so at the rate of 1°F per hour if the environment is warm, but a more usual rate is 1.5–2°F per hour. In this instance the only way of settling the issue was to carry out an unusual investigation – monitoring the temperature in the house by comparing the meteorological readings on the day of her death, 1 May, with those taken some ten days later, and at the same time recording the overnight temperatures of the rooms in the house. Thereby a valid comparison could be made of the approximate loss of heat overnight, providing the meteorological temperatures were not disparate.

I arranged that the temperature in the rear upstairs room (where she was found) the front bedroom and the sitting room downstairs be monitored ten days later from midnight until 8 a.m. It was found that the temperature in the rear upstairs room was maintained at 68°F in all but two hours of the recorded period. Similar readings were given in the front main room and in the lounge. It was therefore clear that the room temperatures we had measured would have been much the same as those at the time of the murder. The weather had been slightly cooler on the date of the killing than it was ten days later but, even so, it was clear that the deceased's rate of body-temperature loss would have been low, of the order of 1°F per hour.

Many pathologists opine that estimating the time of death from temperature measurements is speculative, but it was clear that, owing to the exceptionally warm conditions in the house, the woman's death must have occurred between 11 p.m. the previous night and 3 a.m.

I expected a lengthy cross-examination on this, but the only question I was asked was whether humidity might have played any part in the cooling of the body. The defence team had previously contacted Professor Keith Mant, and he had obviously given them an opinion which was entirely in agreement with my own findings and opinion.

There was some very important circumstantial evidence that pointed at the husband's guilt. First, the taxi cab was noticed to have gone from its parking space by 7 a.m., half an hour earlier than usual, and well before the telephone call he had described. Second, the husband described the television news programme incorrectly. Because of the Chernobyl disaster, there had been unexpected changes. Third, and perhaps most important, the deceased would never have appeared in public without her dentures – she would always have put them in her mouth first thing on getting up. However, her mouth was edentulous at post-mortem examination, and her dentures were found in their usual overnight place in the bathroom cabinet. This was a most damning piece of evidence, since it implied that her death had taken place before the time she would normally have got up in the morning. It seemed certain, taking all this together, that the wife had died either on going to bed or at any rate soon after midnight.

The jewellery on her neck, gripped in order to strangle her, was never found. After death the victim had lain on her back for some hours, and then the accused had dragged her to the spare room, put her spectacles by her and set slippers on her feet. He re-enacted the breakfast scene as though nothing untoward had occurred. It was unfortunate for him that he forgot about the dentures. He was found guilty of murder and sentenced to life imprisonment.

It was Halloween 1981 and a dark, foreboding evening. I sat eyeing some brandy appreciatively after a good dinner, only to be summoned half an hour after midnight to a lonely lane in Hertfordshire, not more than three miles from my home. The reason was a burnt-out car with a body on the back seat, found very near a place known locally as Ridge, owing to its high elevation.

The investigation was triggered by a report from a man at the local RSPCA centre that he had heard an explosion, then seen flames shoot into the night sky. He had called the police, who arrived on the scene prepared to inspect the explosion and fire – which could, of course, have been the result of an accident or a suicidal gesture. An astute WPC noticed some spots of blood on the boot of the car, and these immediately aroused suspicion. A man's body lay across the back seat. The windows had been blown out by the fire, which had been fuelled by petrol from a can which still lay under the driver's seat. On the passenger seat lay a short metal pipe of the type used in scaffolding.

It was soon established that the body was that of the owner of the car, a 45-year-old fishmonger, Michael Walker. He would have been expected at this time of night to be at home with his wife and daughter near St Albans, some seven miles from his fish shop in Potters Bar, north London.

I made a preliminary examination of the body in the car. Because of the awkwardness of getting at it properly, I could hardly make a detailed inspection, but I could see that it was extensively burnt and superficially charred. Later, at Barnet Hospital, I made a thorough examination.

Although there was a small fracture across the back of the skull, the fatal injuries were some six stab wounds in the chest, a couple of which had pierced the heart. There was also a sloping cut on the right cheek, matched by a superficial one on the right shoulder – the cheek wound had passed through the full thickness of the tissue and ended up above his collarbone. There was also a cut on his right leg. These minor injuries had some bearing on his death. It appeared that he had been hit a stunning but not life-threatening blow on the head, probably with the scaffolding pipe. After this he had received a couple of knife wounds. Then, almost certainly as he lay on the ground, a number of stab wounds had been inflicted to his chest, straight into his body without deviation or angulation, delivered by an assailant standing over him.

What was the motive for this unusual murder, and how had the man ended up in a burnt-out car in a remote Hertfordshire lane? Initially the murder appeared to lack a motive, the deceased being a decent honest man with a family and a secure job and background. For several days the police were puzzled. It appeared from the initial investigation that he had met his death outside his house after returning home with the day's takings from his fish shop. His wife, inside, had been unaware as she prepared dinner of the dreadful events unfolding outside. Blood on the forecourt of the house pointed to the stabbing having been perpetrated there, as did evidence of an attempt to disperse the blood with a broom. For some reason the dead man had been driven some five miles in the car to the remote spot where the murderer had attempted to incinerate the body. The explosive nature of the fire was a result of the windows being closed after the petrol was ignited. Some of the day's takings of over £1,000 was found partly burnt in the car, so robbery might not have been the principal motive. Superintendent Reginald Dixon, in charge of the case, thought it was a premeditated attack. Was it some form of revenge killing, possibly associated with the deceased's fondness for greyhound racing?

After patient investigation and inquiries, it emerged that his death was the result of a plan by his wife's lover to kill him and allow her to inherit insurance money to the tune of some £130,000. The connection between the deceased, the wife and the lover became apparent only after the wife, under questioning by police, revealed her lover's name. According to the wife, the plan had been only to apprehend the husband and frighten him into handing over the day's proceeds, the largest of the week. She steadfastly denied that she knew of any plan to murder him. It transpired that the lover and a workmate had collaborated to stab the husband to death following the initial assault, after which the lover drove the body to the lane, the accomplice following in another car.

The two men and the fishmonger's wife were all charged with murder, ostensibly for his money and to enable his wife to continue her association as the accused's mistress. The deceased had known nothing of the liaison.

Members of the public queued for some hours before the start of the trial, such was the local interest. The court and public gallery were packed for the whole two weeks.

As pathologist, I was shown a number of knives. As the wound on the cheek passed in and out of the tissues, it wasn't difficult to gauge the type of knife used, and its length. During the investigation, the wife's lover took police to a canal where a pair of bloodstained trainers and a shotgun cartridge were retrieved. He said he had thrown them there the morning after the murder. It was also the place where a shotgun used to frighten the deceased had been hidden, plus some of the money which had been taken from the car before the fire; however, the knife used for the stabbing was not forthcoming. It is possible that it was a sharp, tapered kitchen knife, as the container for a knife of that type was found in a bedroom wardrobe at the house, its display card bearing the accused's fingerprints.

In addition to my own examination of the deceased, three other pathologists attended on behalf of the defendants for a second examination of the body, but no further opinions were expressed.

As can be surmised, it was a tense, explosive trial. The wife spent a day in the witness box, but her lover, found guilty of her husband's death, did not give evidence. His accomplice did so. The jury took four hours to reach a verdict, clearing the dead man's wife of involvement in the murder and also of an alternative verdict of manslaughter, although she was found guilty of robbery and sentenced to five years. They found the lover guilty of murder, and he was sentenced to life. His accomplice was jailed for nine years for manslaughter and six years for robbery; it was accepted that he had not been the instigator of the robbery, and nor had he planned it, but he had intended to take part in it.

A most unusual development occurred later while the accomplice was serving his time in prison. With the full knowledge of the prison governor, he sent me a letter concerning my views on his involvement in the robbery. He wrote asking about the significance of the blow to the deceased's head, as his prison file did not refer to the fact that it was a lesser injury. The impression given was that he had lashed out at the deceased, a view that might in due course affect his application to the parole board. With the prison governor's permission, I wrote to say that the blow to the head the accomplice had delivered had not been a life-threatening one, although it could have temporarily stunned the victim.

Of all the cases in which it can be difficult to determine whether or not a murder has been committed, those involving battered babies offer the pathologist the greatest problems. The perils and uncertainties of analysing the results of injuries in allegedly battered babies are well known, and there are many instances where it has not been possible to charge a suspected baby batterer, even after a coroner's inquest.

In the relatively early days of the medico-legal investigation of battered babies, before the scenario was widely known outside medical circles, it was difficult to convince a judge or jury of the truth of any such case. These deaths were unexpected and, it was thought, could well have been 'cot deaths' (sudden infant death syndrome). Moreover, it was possible for the defence to suggest a number of medical alternatives to explain any injuries, all of which would have to be excluded by the prosecution during the course of the trial if a successful prosecution was to take place.

In the early 1960s I was called to a south coast town to examine a 2-year-old male child. He was said to have been unwell before collapsing, which he did while he was being washed after a bout of vomiting. His foster-mother had regarded the child as underdeveloped, but visits to the hospital had not confirmed this view. The child had also been in hospital on separate occasions previously with fractures of both upper arms. It was clear from my examination that the child had died after being the subject of gross violence. Not only was the liver ruptured and torn in a number of places, but the supporting tissues of the bowel within the abdominal cavity had also been torn; both these injuries could have occurred only as a result of a violent impact against the abdominal wall or through a powerful and sustained squeeze by a strong arm compressing the child's upper abdomen. As often occurs, there was very little bruising of the abdominal skin. There was also an older injury in the form of a blood clot over the covering of the brain, due to a previous assault.

A powerful force had distorted the normal liver contour, bearing in mind that in a 2-year-old the liver occupies a relatively large part of the abdominal cavity.

In a four-page statement and in evidence to the court at Lewes Assizes, the foster-mother gave a remarkably plausible account of the lad's last day, stating that he had had a convulsion while she was washing his hair in the sink, and that she had summoned help immediately. She added that she had previously been congratulated by the welfare officer on the way she looked after the child, and by the home help. The child's parents, students in London, also complimented the foster-mother on the progress their son was making under her care.

As I listened to her evidence I realized I was going to have a difficult time in the witness box. Once there I explained to the court that the injuries could only have been caused by a fall from a height or a compressive blow to the stomach area. Various suggestions were thrown at me concerning possible causes of these recent injuries. The foster-mother had a back problem, and she said she might have clutched the child to her bosom as she went downstairs from the child's bedroom on the day of the death.

None of these suggestions had any validity, but I do remember the judge looking at me quizzically and asking in all sincerity whether it was really possible that the caring foster-mother whose evidence I had heard could have been responsible for such grievous injuries. Needless to say, the jury was discharged after failing to come to a verdict, and a second trial ensued. At that trial the accused was found not guilty.

I was sorry I had not been more successful in the case on behalf of the Crown, and in particular the Sussex CID, but I was encouraged by reading the opinion for the defence given by Keith Mant. He confirmed my findings, and added that he thought the succession of injuries suffered by children while under this particular foster-mother's care was phenomenal. At least three other children under her care had earlier been badly hurt, including one with two broken legs and a broken arm.

Hindsight indicates that, had more notice been taken of the foster-mother's activities with previous children in her care, and had something been done about it, this death might have been avoided.

Chapter Ten

The Riddle of the Death
of Roberto Calvi

A number of momentous events marked the summer of 1982: the war in the Falklands, the World Cup football competition and on 12 June, Italian television reported the news of the disappearance of Roberto Calvi, chairman of Italy's largest and most important private bank, Banco Ambrosiano, which had close links with the Vatican Bank, the Instituto per le Opere di Religione (IOR). Calvi had left the bank with outstanding loans to the tune of $1.2 billion, mostly irrecoverable and involving subsidiaries as far afield as Panama and Liechtenstein. Rising interest rates and a rising dollar in relation to the Italian lira contributed to the collapse of Banco Ambrosiano following Calvi's disappearance and subsequent death.

Roberto Calvi was born in Milan in 1920, studying at the university there before joining the Italian armed forces during the Second World War, fighting in Russia. Following demobilization, he joined Banco Ambrosiano, founded in 1896. Hardworking and ambitious, he was rapidly promoted, eventually becoming a director and then chairman of the bank. By all accounts, his financial activities increasingly involved the transfer of large sums of money into companies he set up abroad, moving money to offshore investment outlets and later laundering it to make further share purchases in Italy. Calvi had other connections. He was a member of the secret right wing P-2 Masonic Lodge and, reportedly, had links with the Mafia. It all added up to his nickname of God's Banker.

In May 1982 he realized that the bank was in desperate straits. The Bank of Italy was demanding a full account of its activities. He was ousted by fellow directors at a board meeting, following a vote of no confidence.

On 9 June 1982 he left his home in Milan in the company of Flavio Carboni, a Sardinian banker and his close friend. They stayed overnight in Rome, and two days later left for Trieste, where they were joined by one Silvano Vittor. Carboni organized a flight from Trieste to London, and Vittor obtained a false passport for Calvi, whose own had been confiscated the previous year. With companions, the trio arrived at London's Gatwick Airport late on Tuesday 15 June; Calvi's arrival caused no suspicion at passport control. He and Vittor went to Chelsea Cloisters, a block of flats in west London, while the others of their party booked into prestigious accommodation at the London Hilton.

Calvi did not know London at all; perhaps surprisingly, he had no contacts in the City. He shaved off his thin moustache and, as far as can be told, remained closeted in his room, making telephone calls and, no doubt, finding out that the Bank of Italy had taken over Ambrosiano.

On the evening of 17 June, Calvi's last night, Silvano Vittor – who had gone to join those at the Hilton – returned to the apartment and found it locked and empty. Whatever they might have thought had happened to him, over the next two days Calvi's associates left London for Italy.

On the morning of 18 June a City worker, walking along the pedestrian underpass beneath the arches of Blackfriars Bridge, saw the body of a man hanging from scaffolding erected there in connection with some structural work. The police were called and the body was taken to the City of London Mortuary, where Keith Simpson carried out a post-mortem on what was at the time the body of an unknown.

As soon as the identity of the deceased was established, the media were full of the case. I would hear a great deal more about it in later years from the staff of the coroner's court and mortuary where I followed Simpson as pathologist. Although I had no direct involvement with the autopsy, in 1989 I was approached to provide a report on the case for a firm of London solicitors working on behalf of the Italian insurance company Assicurazioni Generali S.p.A. concerning a claim by Calvi's widow on a life assurance policy he held in favour of his family for $4 million.

As noted, Simpson had no idea of the true identity of the man at the time of his examination; the false passport the police had found on the body bore the name Roberto Calvini. Simpson reported that the dead man weighed 13 stone and was wearing a lightweight suit. He found that the lower parts of the trousers were wet and the upper part damp, the former because the trousers had been immersed in water for some time and the latter because it had been drizzling. The deceased was wearing a Patek Phillippe watch. In each jacket and trouser pocket there was a half-brick, and there was also a half-brick down the inside of the trousers between the zip and the underpants. The bricks weighed some 11 pounds in total. The dead man had about him four pairs of spectacles and their cases, twelve wallets, a comb and some 14,000 Swiss francs, plus further cash in Sterling and Italian lira.

Simpson noted that the rope lying loosely around Calvi's neck had a slip knot, and there was a distinctive double line or indentation on the skin surface, rising on each side diagonally upwards and backwards from the front of the neck to a suspension point at the back, between the right ear and the nape of the neck, as seen in cases of suicidal or accidental hanging. Simpson thought the double mark was due to the rope rising or slipping up the neck as the body, partly supported by the water, responded to the varying level of the tide; and he deemed that the appearances were consistent with death by hanging.

On further examination, the rope was found to be some five years old. A distinctive orange colour, it was of a type used for docking boats along the Thames. Calvi might have found it attached to the scaffolding, or he could have obtained it from some other source. (It was later shown indeed to have been left on the scaffolding.)

There was corroborative evidence of hanging in the form of small haemorrhages into the eyelids, though these were not conspicuous. There were no marks of injury to the face, and none of anyone having gripped Calvi by the shoulders or arms; there was no injury to the neck other than the suspension mark, no fracture of the bones of the voicebox. Simpson thought that Calvi's body had dropped two feet before his fall had been partly broken by entry into the water. There were no signs of drowning, so a piece of bone marrow was taken to be examined for the presence of diatoms. (Diatoms are calcified plankton, and are present in large numbers in the Thames water. In cases of drowning they are inhaled in quantity.) These tests were negative, as were tests for drugs.

A small scar on the right thumb and the well marked scar of an older, superficial, self inflicted wound on the undersurface of the right wrist were noticed at the outset by the mortuary staff.

Determining the time of death was obviously an important matter, but temperature recordings were of little value. As rigor mortis was partially complete, it was thought that some eight to twelve hours had elapsed between the death and the examination. The water level of the Thames at the bridge at 2.30 a.m. would not have been high enough to reach Calvi's wrist; conversely, before 1 a.m. the water would have reached his mouth, so that he would have inhaled it and possibly died by drowning rather than hanging. It was deduced, therefore, that he must have died at some time between 1 a.m. and 2.30 a.m. The Patek Phillippe watch, which was not waterproof, had stopped at 1.52 a.m., and this was regarded as a further pointer to the time of death.

A few weeks later, on Friday 23 July, the City of London Coroner, Dr David Paul, held an inquest. The City of London Police had spent many an hour interviewing and collecting information from possible witnesses, but had found nothing whatsoever: no one had noticed Calvi on the night of his death, and there was nothing to show how the man had spent the time following his arrival in London. On examination of his apartment they found suitcases packed, including a toilet kit, all presumably prepared either to leave with him or ready for someone else to collect. A black briefcase that he had had on his arrival in London was not found – although it, or a case just like it, would appear some years later, in 1986, on an Italian television programme.

Unusually, the inquest was taken in one single twelve-hour sitting, with just an hour's break for lunch. In the course of Dr Paul's summing up he mentioned that the jury's tummies must be rumbling after their long day before directing them to the view that a suicide verdict would be right and proper. The jury duly returned that verdict.

In Italy, public opinion was scandalized by the verdict, and Calvi's family incensed, believing he had been murdered. An application was therefore made to a divisional court for the verdict to be quashed, and a second inquest was held the following year under another coroner, Dr Gordon Davies, with George Carman QC representing the family and Richard Du Cann QC appearing for Flavio Carboni, who had not been present or represented at the first inquest.

Carman's brief paid particular attention to the circumstances surrounding Calvi's death and to the possibility that he had been drugged, the suggestion being that the lack of marks of force having been used anywhere on the body might be because he had been subdued or even immobilized by drugs. According to this hypothesis, Calvi could have been overcome by an anaesthetic pad placed over his mouth or, for example, by an injection of curare, which would have paralysed him; a minute injection mark could easily have gone unnoticed at the post-mortem.

Carman pointed out that the circumstances surrounding a death by hanging were as vitally important as the conditions at the subsequent examination, and that in Calvi's case very little was known about those circumstances, other than that there was possible access to the scaffolding either over a wall from the walkway, using a ladder there, or by walking to the scaffolding along the river's edge at low tide. (Simpson had in fact been to the bridge the day after the post-mortem and viewed the scaffolding from the walkway.)

A heavily built man would have had some difficulty moving onto and around the scaffolding, particularly with a half-brick down the front of his trousers and several more half-bricks in his pockets. He would have had to climb over the parapet of the bridge from the walkway and then go down a twelve-foot ladder before stepping over a two-and-a-half-foot gap on to the scaffolding – all this in the very limited light trickling down from the walkway lamps. Indeed the whole operation would have been very awkward for anyone, and doubly so for the brick-encumbered Calvi.

Did he place the bricks in his pockets with the intention of drowning himself by jumping off the scaffolding, but then see the piece of rope and decide to use that instead? This seemed unlikely: it was now known that the rope found around his neck had been tied to the second bar from the top of the scaffolding and attached to a pole at the far end of the structure – well away from the ladder. Again, it was hard to imagine a brick-laden man being able to clamber across to get it, and the notion of him having done so on a sudden whim seemed absurd.

Calvi would have had to stand on the scaffolding, then sit on it while making a slip knot to pass around his neck; he could possibly have made the noose first and then attached the rope to the scaffolding later, but he would have had to be on the scaffolding to carry out this manoeuvre, too.

The alternative explanation – a most sinister one – was that a boat had brought the senseless Calvi to the foot of the scaffolding. Persons unknown could have put the rope around his neck and then hoisted his body to the point of suspension before allowing it to drop. Such an operation would have required more than a holiday dinghy: taking into account the difficulty of manoeuvring on the tideway at that time of night, a powerful motorboat would have been needed. No such boat was ever traced.

Simpson underwent a very vigorous two-hour cross-examination by Carman. The pathologist agreed that, in his vast experience, he had never seen a case of a man hanging whose fall had been broken by water in that manner. He also agreed that he could not exclude the possibility that Calvi had met his death at the hands of other persons. Nevertheless, he did not in any way wish to alter his original opinion as to the cause of death.

The Court had to balance the evidence as to whether it was more likely for a bunch of professional criminals, in a boat with an insensible or petrified Roberto Calvi, to perpetrate a murder, or for Calvi to have taken his own life. The coroner's jury returned an open verdict, which meant that the cause of death was clear but the circumstances surrounding it were unexplained; there was nothing to indicate whether it had been suicide or homicide.

Consider some improbable facts and the background of the case for this having been suicide. Calvi had fled Italy and holed out in a block of flats the other side of London from Blackfriars Bridge. He had chosen to leave his apartment and journey across London – a city he did not know – to the bridge. There was no trace of how he had supposedly made this four-mile journey from Chelsea Cloisters to the bridge late at night. Although in theory it was just possible he could have travelled by London Underground, whose last train arrived at Blackfriars at 1.05 a.m., the bizarreness of his purported actions remains.

In the same year that I was asked to report on the insurance claim, 1989, the international private investigator Kroll Associates reconstructed the incident on behalf of Calvi's son, Carlo. A stand-in was asked to approach the scaffolding, which had been kept in storage, as Calvi might have done, and to clamber over it. Two experienced forensic chemists examined the marks on the loafer shoes worn by the stand-in and compared them with those on the similar shoes Calvi had worn. Traces of yellow paint and rust from the scaffolding poles were clearly evident on the stand-in's shoes; there were no such marks on Calvi's shoes, and this led the chemists to the opinion that Calvi had not walked on the scaffolding unaided. There were, too, no signs of staining or tears on his clothing; furthermore, laser examination suggested that his body had been immersed more deeply in the water than had earlier been appreciated – up to waist-level. This latter finding was a final nail in the coffin of the theory that Calvi could have walked along the river's edge to reach the scaffolding.

In December 1998 Calvi's body was exhumed from the cemetery in Milan, apparently at the request of Flavio Carboni who – with three other men, Franco di Carlo, Pippo Calo and Licio Gelli – had been implicated in causing the death.

Three investigations have taken place since 1982, one involving the City of London Police and the Metropolitan Police, the Kroll Associates investigation in 1989, and, in 1999, an investigation by the pathologist Bernd Brinkman of Munster, Germany. His team, like the Kroll Associates one, concentrated on marks on Calvi's shoes, in this instance scratch marks on the soles at the junction with the heels – an area that does not normally come into contact with the ground. Could these marks be due to Calvi having trampled about on the scaffolding poles? Other, sickle-shaped marks were also found and examined. Indeed, the police photographs of the soles of Calvi's shoes show many scratch marks which are difficult to interpret, in my view – apart from the fact that nobody has mentioned the age of the shoes. According to the Rome newspaper *Il Messaggero* another exhumation of Calvi's body took place in 2002.

It has been alleged that Calvi was met by two Italian men on the night preceding his death, perhaps taken into 'safe custody' and persuaded to board a boat, overcome using drugs, and taken to Blackfriars Bridge, which latter apparently has Masonic connotations.

A similar scenario was depicted in a film based on the case called *I Banchieri di Dio*, (retitled *The Bankers of God* and *God's Bankers* for English-language markets), starring Rutger Hauer. It was given only limited release following an injunction at the request of Flavio Carboni on possible grounds of slander. The film depicts Calvi's death, showing Mafia persons using chloroform to overcome Calvi before strangling him and leaving him hanging from the scaffolding at Blackfriar's Bridge.

A further piece of intriguing information surfaced in October 2002 when a safety deposit box, alleged to have belonged to Calvi, was found in Rome. It came to light in the bank vaults at Nuovo Banco Ambrosiano, the bank set up after the failure of the original one. Although the deposit box had been registered in the names of Calvi and his mother, it was under the control of his brother Leone. The newspaper *La Repubblica* reported that it contained incriminating papers relating to Calvi's death and also part of a brick wrapped in newspaper.

The latest information on the case comes from a panel of judges sitting in Rome who have re-investigated Calvi's death and officially concluded it was murder. Charges are being prepared against four Mafia figures for the crime, Pippo Calo, Flavio Carboni and Manuela Kleinszig, and Ernesto Diotavelli. Under Italian law, the four named have 20 days to present a defence of the Judges' charges. The indictment will go ahead for a trial unless the Judges hear convincing evidence to the contrary.

This latest allegation is based on evidence which has existed for some time, from exhumation examinations which showed that there was no evidence of brick dust on Calvi's hands – which would be present had Calvi used bricks to weight down his body. In addition portions of Calvi's clothing and body fragments including pieces of intestine, tongue and a part of the neck were found in the Milan Institute of Forensic Medicine, presumably relics of the exhumation procedures.

The alleged motive for Calvi's murder is that he mishandled and misappropriated laundered Mafia money. The latter were acting to protect their interests and to prevent blackmail of the P-2 Lodge and Vatican Bank.

Chapter Eleven

Fatal Rioting

The tragic death of PC Keith Blakelock was unique in British forensic history, not only at the time but subsequently, due to proceedings in the civil courts. He was killed during an extremely extensive and violent riot that occurred on the Broadwater Estate, Tottenham, north London. This estate had previously proved a very difficult area to police, and there were frequent outbreaks of violence due to the nature of the buildings. So it proved on the night of Sunday 6 October 1985. The seeds of the riot were events that had taken place the previous day, when Cynthia Jarrett had collapsed and died following a police raid on her house. This occurred because her son had been arrested, incorrectly, for car theft, police deciding to search his mother's house on the premise, also incorrect, that he lived there. Mrs Jarrett was allegedly pushed to the floor.

The subsequent riot in Tottenham lasted most of the night, some five hundred policemen facing a barrage of petrol bombs, bottles and bricks. Machetes, knives and guns were also in evidence. Twenty civilians were injured as well as 223 police officers, seven from gunshot wounds – an often-forgotten aspect of the confrontation between police and rioters. Behind barricades, mobs set cars and buildings alight. All told, 359 persons were arrested, 159 were charged with offences, and, of the 102 cases heard in court, 88 resulted in a conviction or a guilty plea. The use of police photographs taken at the time resulted in 80 persons being identified and, directly, to 40 pleas of guilty, the offences involved ranging from threatening behaviour to affray, riot and, finally, murder.

The disturbance came to a climax with the assault involving PC Blakelock, who collapsed after sustaining several blows from a variety of weapons. Blakelock had been part of a team of twelve officers sent into a section of the estate to escort and protect firemen who were attempting to put out a fire in a supermarket. It was a difficult situation, due to the buildings and their stairways. As a group of officers retreated down a narrow stairwell they became the target of missiles and petrol bombs. It was subsequently alleged that there was mishandling of the operation by the police, the estate not being kept under police surveillance and there being insufficient backup by police officers. One officer attested to the riot being led, in his opinion, by a masked man brandishing a machete, and he saw Blakelock being attacked as he lay on the ground. Those officers who were repeatedly struck by implements doubted they could escape with their lives, particularly those on the staircase – indeed, some of the rioters chanted exactly this, that the policemen would not get out alive.

An officer tried to drag Blakelock to safety and, with another officer's help, got him to the police lines, a knife protruding from the side of his neck.

The day following the riot I met Detective Chief Superintendent Graham Melvin, in charge of the inquiry. My examination of the body required a careful appraisal of the many wounds Blakelock had sustained. They were unusual due to their number and the differing pattern of injuries. So horrific were the wounds that at the trial the judge directed that the jury should not see photographs. Blakelock had been found lying prone, so almost all the wounds were on the back of his body, except for some protective wounds on the hands and arms sustained before he collapsed, attempting to ward off blows from his assailants. There were thirteen wounds on the back, mostly superficial, clearly caused by the point or blade of a sharp knife entering the tissues. There were eight head wounds, chiefly on the left side, but no fracture of the skull. Some of the head wounds had been caused by a curved weapon, probably metal, some by a sharp knife-like weapon. There were superficial wounds on the face, which could have been due to a knife with a hooked, notched or serrated edge, and there was a massive wound inflicted by a weapon like an axe or machete across the right side of the neck, gaping in appearance, which had fractured the lower jawbone and passed through all the soft tissues.

The most dramatic and horrendous injury involved the knife which protruded from the back of the right side of his neck. It went six inches deep into the tissues to reach the back of the mouth, close to the spinal column.

There were other injuries of a different type, notably on the shoulders, caused by stamping, but nothing of significance on the legs or front of the body.

In all, there were forty stabbing or cutting injuries. The only question I was asked in cross-examination was to confirm that the serious injuries were confined to the back of the body and occurred after the officer had collapsed to the ground.

The CID had conducted a very difficult investigation – as had I, of course, in assessing whether the wounds had been caused by a specific weapon. From the police angle, any information from my examination might help them and lead to charges against suspects or those arrested. In an attempt to correlate wounds with weapons, over the subsequent weeks I was presented with a number of weapons, including a clasp knife, a five-inch-long serrated knife, a single-bladed knife some six inches long and one inch wide, and a sheath knife. Examination was made by comparison of the measurements with those of the wounds. The clasp knife was possible for some wounds but other weapons did not entirely fit the bill. I also examined an electric heating element which could have caused the head wounds. It was impossible to identify any specific weapon as having caused the injuries I found; there must have been other weapons which had been removed from the scene.

In the event, six persons were charged with murdering Blakelock and sent for trial at the Central Criminal Court, the trial lasting for three months in the first part of 1987. The accused included three juveniles who were cleared at the direction of the judge, who said the police had been guilty of being burdensome, harsh, wrongful and unjust in their handling of the trio.

The adult man accused and charged with Blakelock's murder was Winston Silcott, who was said to have hacked the officer to death. He was found guilty and jailed for life, with the recommendation that he remain in prison for thirty years. Subsequently his conviction was quashed. The two youths charged with him, Mark Braithwaite and Engin Raghip, also had their convictions quashed.

Winston Silcott's successful appeal in November 1991 against his conviction was based on forensic scientists' examination of police notes in relation to fabricated evidence. His advisers pursued claims for wrongful imprisonment and he was awarded £17,000 compensation from the Home Office. This action was followed by one against the Commissioner of the Metropolitan Police on grounds of false imprisonment and malicious prosecution, resulting in an award of £50,000 in November 1999, some fourteen years after Blakelock's death, at a time while Silcott was in prison serving a life sentence for a separate murder conviction. In 1989 an independent inquiry headed by Lord Gifford had criticized police handling of the case.

Blair Peach's death followed a fierce confrontation between

police and protestors in Southall, London, in April 1979. It evolved from a National Front rally on 23 April, prior to that year's General Election. The cornerstone of the National Front's manifesto was compulsory repatriation of immigrants. Not unnaturally, community leaders in the area were dismayed that the rally had been permitted to take place, particularly in Southall, where a substantial proportion of the population was of Asian or West Indian origin.

The Anti-Nazi League had been organized to oppose National Front meetings all over the country and they mounted a counter-rally. The third party involved were two units of the Special Patrol Group of police officers, an elite mobile reserve deployed at demonstrations, terrorist sieges and scenes of public disorder. A call for assistance came from No. 3 Unit of the SPG when its contingent was pelted with bottles and bricks after leaving their vehicles to deal with and arrest persons throwing stones. By the end of the day a total of 2,800 police officers would be involved; there were 342 arrests, and 97 police officers were injured in addition to a similar number of civilians.

Everything pointed towards a violent demonstration. Hundreds of Asians had assembled in Southall Broadway, together with many young white people including many members of the Anti-Nazi League. People came from all parts of London, among them Blair Peach, aged 33, originally from New Zealand but a UK resident for a decade or so working as a teacher in the East End of London. He had joined the Anti-Nazi League and the Socialist Workers' Party, becoming a leading militant.

Police tactics were to keep separate the two factions of demonstrators – the National Front and their opponents – but nevertheless there were scuffles in the Broadway, near the Town Hall. Officers were hit by stones and police subsequently pursued the demonstrators with truncheons, extending their activities down alleys and into gardens.

It was at this point in time that Blair Peach was fatally injured, struck on the head by some implement, the identity of which became the subject of considerable conjecture. Found sitting wounded on the pavement, he was helped into an adjacent house, and just after 8 p.m. an ambulance arrived, taking him to nearby Ealing Hospital.

At the hospital Peach was found to have sustained a head injury which had resulted in extensive fragmentation of the bone of the side of his head, resulting in tearing of an artery whose branches fan out on the inner table of the skull, between the bone and the brain coverings. Despite attempts to relieve the pressure of blood accumulating within the cranial cavity and the efforts of a senior surgeon, Peach died close on midnight. The stage was set for a post-mortem and an inquest.

A feature of this head injury was the fact that, apart from the bruising in the scalp tissues adjacent to the fracture, there was no sign of injury to the skin surface, a most unusual finding. There was a wide area of bone missing from the left side of the top of the skull, having been removed during surgery, but the original fracture line could be seen extending across the midline of the top of the skull, entering the base of the skull on the other side. I confirmed the main fracture running through the branches of the artery, and I also examined fragments of bone preserved from the operation.

It was evident that the thickness of the skull was not entirely normal, and later I confirmed that it was thinner than one would expect in a man of this age. Instead of a quarter-inch thick at its thickest point, three-sixteenths of an inch for most of the rest and one-eighth of an inch at the thinnest point (which is at the side of the head just above the lobe of the ear), the first two readings were three-sixteenths and one-eighth of an inch respectively; the thinnest point was less than one-sixteenth of an inch thick. This could be of importance in relation to determining the effect of a blow against the side of the head, as the internal damage would be considerably greater than with a normal skull.

Would it have made any difference to the final outcome? I wonder if the explanation for there being no injury to the skin was that the blow was insufficient to cause skin injury but sufficient for the transmitted impact to cause the skull fracture. The multiple fracture of the skull meant that bleeding from several arterial branches had occurred, and this would have caused rapid unconsciousness and pressure on the underlying brain.

Subsequently the Friends of Blair Peach Committee was founded, some £20,000 was raised for their campaign – which included the display of posters naming SPG officers 'WANTED FOR MURDER' – and a record, *The Murder of Blair Peach*, was made.

A second post-mortem was carried out on behalf of the Blair Peach family, Keith Mant from Guy's Hospital coming to a similar conclusion to my own. Rufus Crompton from St George's Hospital, Tooting, with experience as a neuro-pathologist, also examined the deceased but had no significant alternative conclusions to bring in evidence, although later he said he thought the blow that caused Blair Peach's death could have been from a truncheon wielded so that it crushed the skin so quickly as not to split it. My view was that the injury was caused not by a truncheon but possibly by a police radio set.

I examined a number of items and implements taken from lockers of officers in the SPG, including a riot shield, a short standard police truncheon, an eight-inch police truncheon and the handle of a rhino whip; also an American night stick, a couple of jemmies, the wooden handle of a hammer, a wooden stave with a leather covering, jack handles, a ribbed wooden truncheon, a lead cosh and the favoured radio, measuring seven inches by three inches by two inches and weighing over a pound. I excluded all the other weapons found, as they would likely have caused laceration of the scalp. Needless to say, most of the weapons I examined should not have been available to police officers.

The inquest opened in Fulham Town Hall in October 1979, but was adjourned as no jury was present. Counsel for the Peach family maintained that a jury should be summoned, on the grounds that the inquest related to circumstances which could be prejudicial to public safety. The coroner, Dr John Burton, rejected that view, stating that Parliament had amended the law so that a jury did not have to be called in such a situation. The argument was eventually resolved, and the inquest was resumed at Hammersmith Coroner's Court in May 1980 with a jury of five men and four women, who heard evidence from some eighty-four witnesses.

Hammersmith Coroner's Court has seen many important inquests in its time. Over eighteen days about seventy persons were crammed into the small courtroom. There was a remarkable diversity of witnesses' accounts as to events surrounding Blair Peach's death. Some claimed he was hit by one officer, others by more than one, and some gave similar accounts regarding the activities of a different officer. There were varying opinions expressed as to how many times Blair Peach was hit, and even where he was at the time it occurred; none of the witnesses could give a detailed description of the officers involved, and no one had been picked out at identification parades held for that purpose.

It was unfortunate that at the inquest only the coroner and the counsel for the Metropolitan Police had copies of all the statements and of a report of a police inquiry that had taken place into Peach's death. This fact probably hampered counsel for the participating parties, particularly the Peach family, the Anti-Nazi League and the Police Federation, although the coroner hastened to reveal anything from those reports he thought material to his inquiry.

Even so, the DPP had previously decided there was

insufficient evidence to justify proceedings against any officer – although four officers of the SPG were transferred to other duties.

Summing up, Dr Burton told the jury that, if they considered a riot had taken place and if in their view the police used reasonable force in the execution of their duties – Peach being one of the rioters – they should return a verdict of misadventure. Such a verdict was also reasonable if Peach had been hit by a police officer who was chasing another person involved in the riot. But, if the jury believed Peach had been deliberately killed while acting lawfully, the verdict would be unlawful killing. The jury added two riders to their verdict of accidental death – first, that in such events the SPG should be more strictly controlled and have better liaison with local police, and, second, that no unauthorized weapons should be available to or carried by police officers. (In fact, riders are not valid at inquests, though juries may make recommendations.)

Following these events the role of the SPG altered greatly, and the Home Secretary of the day, William Whitelaw, decided that the service of SPG officers should be limited to four years, that more supervising officers should be included, and that the unit should be decentralized to individual Metropolitan Police areas. The Special Patrol Group does not exist any longer.

Rioting always has a cause. It could be that the Broadwater Estate riots stemmed from the preceding police presence in Mrs Jarrett's home, and her consequent death. These circumstances were not dissimilar to the ones pertaining in 1985 when the south London flat of Dorothy Groce was raided by police. Both areas had a multicultural community.

On 28 September 1985, during a security operation in Brixton, Mrs Groce's flat was raided, ostensibly with the aim of questioning her son Michael, in connection with a robbery that had occurred in Hertfordshire. Inspector Douglas Lovelock, a qualified marksman who was armed, and three officers went inside the house. Mrs Groce, generally known as Cheri, had been sleeping downstairs; her husband and younger son were also present in the room. While lying in bed, at about 7 a.m., she heard noises in the hallway and, thinking it might be her daughter, she went to the bedroom door – just as it was thrown open, pushing her backwards. Police officers rushed in, one holding a small gun. She felt a pain in her left shoulder, heard a bang and realized she had been shot. She collapsed.

Mrs Groce did not see which officer was responsible for the shooting, but the bullet from the gun held by Inspector Lovelock was found embedded in the wall of the bedroom, having passed through her body. The wound caused permanent paralysis from the waist downwards. She was taken to St Thomas's Hospital and subsequently Stoke Mandeville Hospital, Aylesbury, for further treatment.

This incident was followed by a most serious riot, one of the worst in the country for years. To raise tempers yet higher, a rumour had circulated that Mrs Groce had been shot twice – a misinterpretation of the fact that there were two wounds on her body, the entrance and exit wounds of a single bullet.

Hugh Johnson, who examined Mrs Groce in St Thomas's several days after the shooting and prepared his report, died a short time later, and I was asked to examine documents relating to the court case that followed.

Mrs Groce, five feet tall, had received a firearm wound on the upper part of the left side of the chest, producing a typical entry wound. The bullet had travelled in a downwards direction after entering the body, and from left to right, passing through the chest and the spine and making its exit on the right side of her back, close to the midline.

I accordingly gave evidence at the trial of Inspector Lovelock at the Central Criminal Court, Old Bailey. The pressure required to pull the trigger of the Smith and Wesson revolver was an

important part of the case against Lovelock, and I was questioned on his reaction to the stress and tension in the situation he
faced. I thought that tension in his muscles at the time of the
incident would increase during the initial entry and confrontation in the flat, and I also considered that his state of mind could
have affected his physical reaction: if he had consciously
attempted to overcome such stress, tension in his muscles might
increase. The inference was that the inspector was more likely
to have pulled the trigger when under severe mental and
physical stress. Of course, such views are not usually given as
evidence by a forensic pathologist, but here I was speaking as a
doctor generally. The passage of the bullet through the body
was consistent with the victim having been in a semi-crouching
position at the time.

The upshot was that Inspector Lovelock, an officer for
twenty-one years and previously commended for bravery, was
found not guilty by the jury but had to appear before the Police
Complaints Authority. Mrs Groce received compensation for
the injury, which had left her paralysed for the rest of her life.

Chapter Twelve

Unsolved Murders

Unsolved murders are the bane of a detective's life, and cause heartache to the victim's relatives and friends. They receive more than usual publicity, partly due to media interest, increased when the CID make available details and information about the case which could result in a prosecution. Fortunately, the percentage of unsolved murders is relatively small, although clearly true incidence is not known because undetected homicides, by definition, cannot be added to the statistics.

Murders where a sexual attack takes place away from home and family, or in circumstances where the person responsible is unknown to the victim, or where both parties are known to each other but friends and colleagues do not know of the relationship or friendship, are difficult to solve. Such instances are often rooted in a sexual liaison, perhaps with jealousy or revenge as a predominant factor. Other examples are the tragic cases of child murder, where paedophiles may operate as serial killers; and homicides for which there is no obvious motive. The latter present the hardest of all investigations. Their fascination is that they are usually remembered for many years afterwards, even though the passage of time may not lead to any new evidence.

A number of unsolved murders illustrate the difficulty.

The year following my appointment at Charing Cross Hospital Medical School, I was called to Southgate, north London, where a 26-year-old French au pair girl, Odette du Mourier, had been found lying in the front garden of a house at a road junction shortly after midnight. She was taken to a nearby hospital and pronounced dead. It was the height of summer and I was summoned at 5 a.m. to examine the scene – a vital part of any such inquiry but one sometimes overlooked through the police or, worse still, the pathologist not thinking it necessary. At the scene I met one of the finest and most perceptive detectives it has been my privilege to meet, Detective Superintendent Sidney Bradbury, a remarkable man. No investigation was considered too small or too insignificant for him to oversee, particularly at the scene. A thoughtful and intelligent detective, he usually spotted clues in a murder inquiry which others might have missed.

The site where the body was found told me nothing, but I was put into the picture as to the nature of the crime and, after a preliminary examination, conducted a full examination in the hospital mortuary. This was an important case for me to handle at this stage of my career, and any slipshod investigation, casual manner or mistake would be noted by Bradbury and his team for future reference. There were other pathologists in the area equally capable and probably more experienced than I was.

The girl had been working as an au pair and had been out for the evening with a boyfriend, who had to hurry to catch his last train home instead of escorting her, as was his custom, to the nearby house where she lived. A passing motorist, seeing the girl's handbag lying on the pavement, had stopped and taken it to the local police station. The boyfriend was excluded from the investigation after inquiries.

There had been up to twelve attacks relatively recently on women within a six-mile radius of where Odette was found, all fortunately non-fatal – though it is not infrequent, when a death of this nature occurs, that previously forgotten incidents are recalled. It seemed that these assaults had followed a similar pattern: the attacker lurked in the shadows waiting to pounce on an unsuspecting girl as she walked home from the underground station late at night.

The deceased girl had received three blows to the front of her head, leaving lacerated wounds but no fracture of the underlying skull, two blows on the left side of the head and five on the back of the head, the main one of which latter had fractured the skull. These were very serious multiple injuries. There were also minor injuries to the arms and legs, including one to the hand, the latter probably protective in nature as she had tried to ward off a blow. The main injuries to the head had caused a fatal internal haemorrhage around the brain. There were also, significantly, some fine linear grazes around the groin due to her knickers having been forcibly pulled upwards as she lay prone on the ground, but otherwise there was no evidence of sexual interference or assault. The assailant had probably been disturbed by the passing motorist, the attack occurring at about 11.30 p.m.

A search was made for the weapon used. The pattern of injury suggested she had been attacked initially from the front, then, as she fell or as she lay on the ground, further blows – more severe ones – had been inflicted on the back of the head. The detectives were looking for a blunt instrument – a piece of piping or some form of spanner. An Army bomb-disposal unit was brought in and used metal detectors to search in a wide area, but all in vain. Some two months later I was shown three metal tools, including a spanner, which might have been used in the attack.

This murder in a pleasant suburb caused considerable apprehension in the community. The CID investigated the possibility that the girl had been followed in the week before her death, and house-to-house inquiries were made. A man in his thirties had been seen in the road a short time before Odette started walking home, but he could not be linked with any of the previous attacks reported. Bradbury left no stone unturned in his team's investigation, but all without success.

Following a case of this nature, the coroner opens an inquest as to the cause of death, and later, after a trial, the result is reported back to the coroner, who only then closes the inquest. In an unsolved murder, the coroner holds a full inquest attended by all witnesses, and a verdict of unlawful killing is usually given against person or persons unknown. Curiously enough, years ago it was the practice that an initial murder inquiry was heard in the coroner's court before the case reached the criminal court. The procedure may also start in a coroner's court if the Director of Public Prosecutions does not feel there is initially sufficient evidence for the case to go to the magistrates' or crown court.

One becomes inured to most scenes of crime, just as a surgeon is oblivious of the instruments, retractors, pulsating arteries, glistening organs and haemorrhage in the course of his theatre work. Pathologists can cope with scenes of murder as at the time of the examination they are preoccupied with the details, but occasionally an investigating officer finds it too stressful, as in the following case.

One visits scenes of crime from waste ground to mansions. In this 1974 case the setting was akin to an Agatha Christie mystery. The house the deceased occupied, standing well back from the road in Hadley Green, north London, was some 200 yards away from her childhood home. It was a substantial detached house with a splendid garden and a through driveway in front, with a number of French windows overlooking the garden. There were four bedrooms as well as an attic room. The occupant, a 57-year-old widow named Mrs Stephanie Britton, had lived all her life in the area – baptism, marriage and, alas, funeral all taking place in the local parish church.

On a bitterly cold Saturday morning, 12 January, I met Detective Superintendent Perkins at the scene. He had a long experience of investigating crimes of all sorts, but he was not prepared for the scene which confronted him – so much so that, after the initial investigation, he decided it would be better if he were replaced by another officer. In the threshold of the sitting room, close to the doorway which led to the hall and front door, lay Mrs Britton's body, fully clothed. Her spectacles were just within the hallway. She had been sitting in a comfortable armchair a short distance (some six to eight feet) from the hall; an open book lay between the arm and seat of the chair, and there were two mugs on an adjacent table. The daily paper was on the back of the chair. There was no sign of a struggle or any disturbance of the contents of the room – in contrast to the disorder found elsewhere in the house. The room was cold, the body, by the time I got to it, was approaching room temperature at 63°F, so it was possible to estimate only a very approximate time of death. Although this was a sharp January morning, the deceased had been economical with the heating in the house owing to a power crisis. The curtains in the room were closed. There was no disturbance of the deceased's clothing, but some cuts to the face were apparent, with bloodstains on her pullover.

Upstairs, in the bedroom overlooking the front of the house, the body of a small child, her grandson, lay in pyjamas, half in and half out of bed, one arm extending to the floor, blood dried on his face and the floor and blood staining his pyjama jacket and bedclothes. A chest of drawers had been pulled out and the contents strewn in a haphazard manner on the floor. The rooms upstairs had been ransacked, the disturbance too formal to be genuine. Nothing of value had been taken – antiques or jewellery.

Later examination showed that the injuries which had caused both deaths were almost identical in nature. The grandmother had sustained a number of stab wounds, nine in all, five piercing and causing injuries and haemorrhage to the lungs and heart, clearly caused by a knife with a blade one inch wide and at least six inches long and having a single sharp edge. There were a couple of superficial injuries on the back of the body. The facial and head injuries were due to kicking or stamping blows from a shod foot.

The boy's injuries to the chest and back were similar to his grandmother's, causing fatal haemorrhage. There were no other injuries or signs of a struggle.

The front door had been bolted inside, but one of the french windows had been found open by the boy's mother, who had arrived earlier that morning to discover the tragedy.

It was clearly a bizarre double murder, a situation not unlike a fictional mystery. To add to this impression, a distinctive carving knife was missing from the cutlery drawer.

It was all most puzzling: no apparent break-in, the deceased disturbed from her reading and cruelly murdered, and likewise her grandson upstairs. As the newspapers commented, there was no obvious motive – sexual assault or robbery. These two defenceless persons, in the quiet of the evening, had been done to death, the motive known only to the person responsible.

The coroner's inquest some months later got no further with the murder inquiry, although some background information came to light. The deceased lady's daughter (the mother of the boy stabbed to death) was separated from her husband, and her boy, four years old, had been taken to stay overnight with his grandmother, Mrs Britton, who was expected to return the child to his mother the following morning. When this did not occur and the daughter received no reply to a telephone call, she went to the house, found it in darkness with no signs of an intruder, and discovered her mother as I have described. The only other witness at the inquest, the deceased's sister, had received a telephone call from Mrs Britton at about 10.30 p.m. the previous evening, cancelling some arrangements. Mrs Britton must have met her death sometime shortly afterwards.

No arrest was ever made. Looking back it seems that the deceased must have welcomed or at least admitted somebody known to her into the house, and that this somebody subsequently stabbed her and her grandson. Four years later a knife with its handle missing was found on the nearby common. Its measurements were consistent with the wounds I had examined, but there the matter rested. Even the hardened and experienced Detective Chief Superintendent William 'Tug' Wilson, a top Scotland Yard Murder Squad detective, said it was one of the worst murders he had encountered.

Who knows? This crime may arouse thoughts and memories and a guilty conscience in someone, even after the passage of twenty-eight years.

A popular general practitioner in Amersham, Buckinghamshire, Dr Helen Davidson had practised there for twenty-one years, retaining her maiden name for professional purposes. Set in the heart of the county, Amersham has a charmingly picturesque old high street and the surrounding conurbation is well built, largely a farming community with fields surrounding the town. The doctor, 54 years old, had married late in life to a bank official some twenty years her senior, the marriage taking place some six years prior to her murder.

On the day of her death, 9 November 1966, she left her home in Chesham Bois, a village just to the north of Amersham, shortly after 1.30 p.m., her husband having departed earlier for Chesham, another local village, where he did some part-time work. It was a lovely late autumn afternoon and she evidently had decided to take a walk with her dog, Fancy. Well clothed, with a raincoat over outdoor walking clothing, and with a dog chain in one of her pockets, she set out, bypassing Amersham, the walk taking her to Hodgemoor Wood, some two miles away.

She was a bird watcher, and took her binoculars. She did not return home, and an overnight search proved fruitless. The following afternoon her body was found in Hodgemoor Wood, a short distance from the main Amersham to Beaconsfield road.

She lay on her back, fully dressed, with no signs of interference of her clothing, the collar and sleeves of her nylon raincoat blood-spattered and the outdoor gloves she was wearing heavily bloodstained. The binocular strap was around her neck, the binoculars between her head and right shoulder. Her dog, Fancy, lay curled up between her legs, uninjured.

I was called by the Buckinghamshire CID to meet Detective Chief Superintendent Barker and two Detective Chief Inspectors, Barrett and Napier, the latter from Scotland Yard, at the wood at 7.45 p.m. that evening. My secretary and I drove to Stockings Farm at the edge of the wood, a large U-shaped area some mile by half a mile in extent, crossed by footpaths and bridleways. We walked into the wood, where I was shown the deceased. Rigor mortis was established, indicating that death had occurred at least twenty-four hours before she was found; temperature readings were valueless so far as time of death was concerned. There was a very extensive and severe wound across the upper half of her face, with a dark deposit around its margins, a finding of some significance. I had never encountered such a case.

Later that evening at the local hospital I carried out an examination, joined by Detective Superintendent Jack 'Razor' Williams from the Murder Squad, Scotland Yard, who had, as the papers put it, 'been called in'. Williams was a forthright character and just the man to investigate such a murder, which he did with energy but also with tact and expediency.

As I suspected from my initial examination, the severe wound across the left side of the face had obliterated the eye, extending to the base of the skull, causing extensive fractures of the bones around the left eye, including the upper jaw and nose. There was

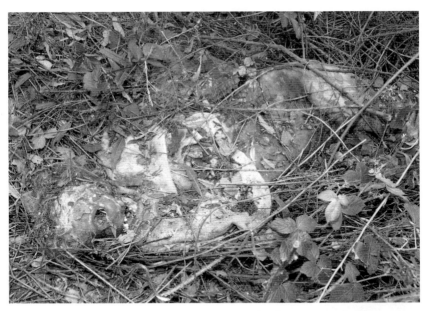

Site of discovery of body near railway embankment, Hertfordshire.

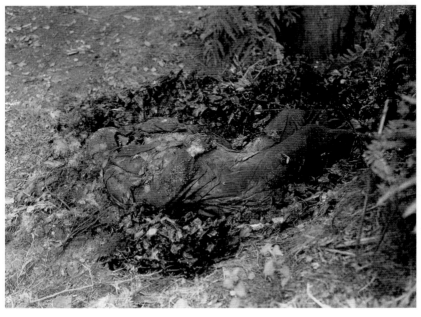

Peter Thomas's body in shallow grave adjacent to
country road, Bracknell, Berkshire.

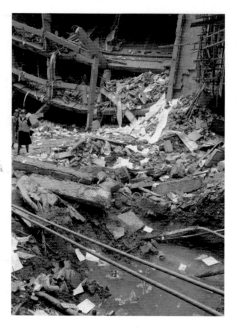

The Chamber of Shipping building, St Mary Axe, in the City of London after an IRA bomb.

Aircraft crash at Heathrow, London; overturned fuselage adjacent to passenger terminal.

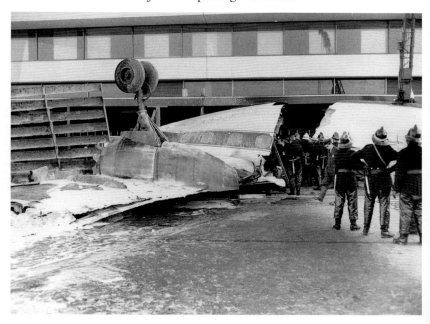

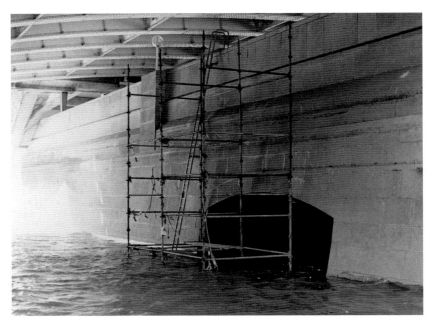

Scaffolding at Blackfriars Bridge, London, where Calvi's body was found.

Passport found in Calvi's clothing.

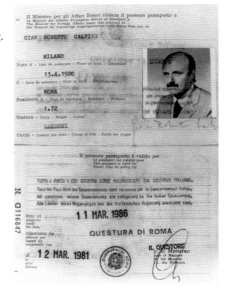

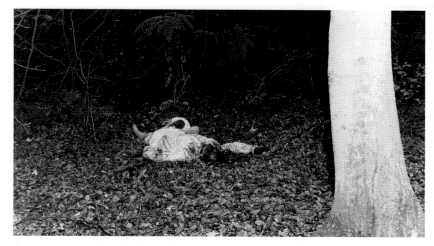

Unsolved murder, Amersham, Buckinghamshire.
Deceased with dog resting on her legs.

Moundis, the man accused of
Ann Chapman's murder.

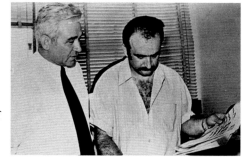

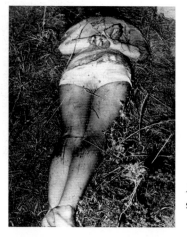

Ann Chapman's body in a
sheep fold near Athens.

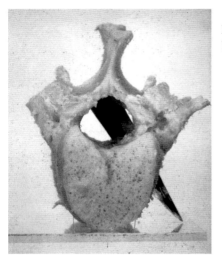

Broken knife blade through vertebral body following a stab wound.

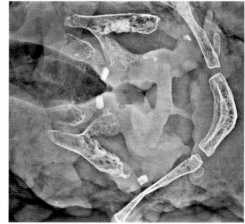

Fracture of bone in larynx from strangulation case where the tiny bone is bent.

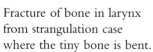

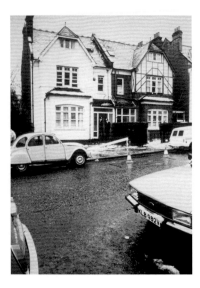

Nilsen's flat on the top floor of the house at Cranley Gardens, north London.

Manhole with cover removed at Cranley Gardens; site of discovery of human remains.

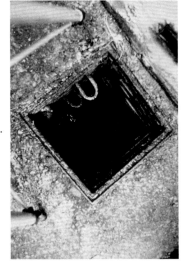

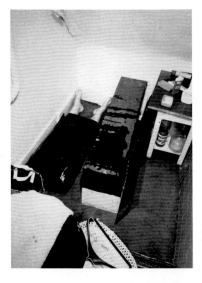

Nilsen's bathroom at Cranley Gardens. Wall bench removed to show body.

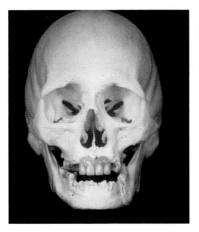

Skull of Nilsen's penultimate victim at Cranley Gardens showing healed fracture of jaw and denture.

Incinerated bone fragments from Nilsen's garden at Melrose Avenue, north London.

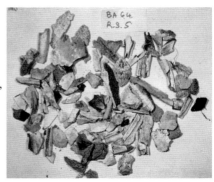

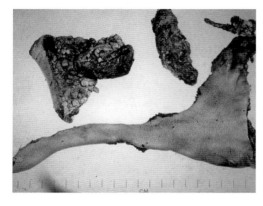

Pieces of skin removed from manhole, brought to author for examination.

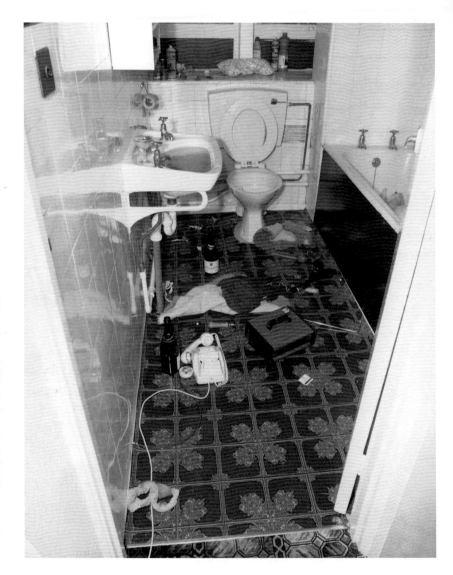

Belan case; bathroom with body in bath.

a wound of similar type, but this time superficial, across the skin of the forehead, and there were minor injuries to the lower lip and chin, possibly due to blows from a foot. The margins of the main wound were contaminated by the dark, almost granular material I had noticed on the face at the scene. Examined in the laboratory, the material proved to be charcoal.

A large piece of burnt wood found at the scene gave a positive test for blood on its surface, and was almost certainly the murder weapon. The woods had been the subject of tree thinning, and presumably some of the waste wood had been burnt; the bloodstained piece of wood probably came from an old bonfire. It must clearly have been wielded with tremendous force: when the deceased was removed from the scene there was a three-inch-deep indentation in the undergrowth behind and beneath her head.

One further piece of information came from the autopsy. The stomach was half full of food, in keeping with her death having been within four hours or so of a meal being taken. This suggested death at about 4 p.m. the previous day, just before it became dark.

It was clear that tracing the assailant would pose a problem. First, motive – or lack of it. It was highly unlikely that the doctor went to the wood to meet someone. It may well have been that, while out walking through the wood that November afternoon, she recognized someone who had no business to be there. Could she have been mistaken for a private detective, with her binoculars? – in which case a courting couple or secret lovers might have feared exposure.

In any event, she had been viciously bludgeoned to death with a piece of wood, the only implement to hand at the time. The fact that the blow had obliterated the upper face and eyes could be of significance, as could be that her binoculars had been stamped upon. As 'Razor' Williams said, it might have been the binoculars that led to her death. She had, as far as was known, no enemies in the village or her practice, and it was improbable that she would have been followed to the wood for a premeditated attack.

At the subsequent inquest I gave evidence that there was no sexual assault, and no obvious attempt by Dr Davidson to defend herself. The blow which bludgeoned her to death was almost certainly caused by a person who knew the locality. Some 2,000 people were interviewed during the inquiry and some 1,000 statements taken. If only her dog, Fancy, could have talked. Once more, somebody's conscience may still be tormented by those horrifying events of thirty-six years ago.

Women walking alone or living on their own may be more susceptible to criminal attacks – usually sexual – than other persons in the community, and the same applies to those who work on their own, such as the middle-aged woman Sylvia Taylor who was the manager of a licensed shop in Brighton in the mid-1960s when she was murdered.

I went down in May 1965 to meet Detective Chief Superintendent John Marshall, a good-humoured and astute detective who kept a close eye on criminal activities in his jurisdiction. The deceased lay in the corner of the back office of the shop, on her back, her arms at her side, legs bent at the knees. She was fully clothed except for her left breast, which was exposed, where the clothing had been clearly pulled down on to the arm and lower chest. Her skirt was drawn upwards on to her hips, but there was no obvious disturbance of her knickers. On a desk nearby were her spectacles. There was no sign of a struggle. After making various temperature measurements, I came to the conclusion, seemingly confidently, that her death had occurred between 6 p.m. and 8 p.m. the previous evening. Looking back now, I was confining her death to a very narrow interval of time – against good practice but, by chance, in this instance remarkably accurate.

My examination showed the characteristic marks of manual strangulation on her neck and, in particular, indented fingernail abrasions on her mouth, chin and, more definitely, her neck. This view was supported by asphyxial changes in the face, all due to constriction of the neck and the damming up of blood in the facial tissues. There was no damage to the voicebox but the findings were consistent with the deceased having been gripped firmly by a right hand, the thumb on the lower part of the neck on the left side and the fingers on the opposite side, high up and around the mouth. But an adjacent heavy steel safe was open – although nothing appeared to be missing. It was a mysterious death.

It transpired that a man had called at the off-licence at 6.20 p.m. to purchase some whisky, setting a limit to how early she might have been murdered. The body was found at 9.40 p.m. by a passer-by who saw the small cardboard sign on the front door indicating the shop was open. It surprised him that the shop should be open so much later than usual, so he went inside – and discovered the unwelcome scene. But who was responsible? It was certainly no one in her family, as they were all traced and their activities that day accounted for; and the deceased appeared from all reports to have been a sensible business-woman with nothing untoward in her private life. We can only assume that a customer entered the shop – perhaps he knew her, rather than vice versa – possibly decided to proposition her, was rejected, and strangled her.

The coroner returned an open verdict – one of murder by person or persons unknown would have been more appropriate as of course we knew the cause of death: she had been strangled.

I have had my share of unsolved murders, although probably no more than my colleagues. But one case in particular came back to me and to the notice of the police some years after it had occurred. No trial or conviction had taken place.

A 14-year-old schoolgirl, Joyce Morris, left school early, at midday, on 19 June 1980, and was last seen at about 12.15 p.m. near the back door of her home in West Middlesex. It was raining heavily and when seen she appeared to be soaking wet. She could not gain entrance to her home without a door key, so she went off somewhere – it was thought she was making her way to meet her parents. She had left school early on some six previous occasions earlier that year for no apparent reason, but this time when she did not return home she was reported missing.

Her body was found some two days later and I made an examination at the scene – an area adjacent to the historic airfield at Heston, where Neville Chamberlain landed from Munich with his famous 'piece of paper' after his meeting with Adolf Hitler in 1938.

The girl lay face-down next to a pathway across the heath, well surrounded by undergrowth, which consisted of tall bamboo-like canes. She was fully clothed, although her tights and two pairs of pants were around her ankles. Her satchel lay at the side of her body, one of its straps running through the fingers of her left hand and around her right wrist. She was wearing a pullover, grey shirt, blue skirt and belt, and a slip. Her high-heeled shoes were covered in earth on the undersurface between the heel and the sole, and there was some dirt staining on her feet.

Her hands had been tied together in front of her body with a pair of tights using three loops around both wrists; reddish pressure marking of the skin indicated firm contact with the material. Her death was due to a ligature – a pair of tights completely encircling the neck had deeply indented the skin and caused intense asphyxial changes.

Rigor mortis tests indicated she had been dead for some 36–48 hours prior to my examination, so she had been strangled sometime on the day of her disappearance, but there was no more accurate means of assessing the time of death. There were many other puzzling points concerning her death. Here was a girl leaving school at lunchtime on the first day of the week, for no good stated reason, found dead some way from her home, close to open heath land. Had she met someone by appointment or arrangement? Had things gone wrong, or had it been a strangulation on impulse, carried out by an unknown stranger? Did it occur in the undergrowth where she was found or in the open, her body being carried to its resting-place? There was no sign of sexual interference other than her pants and tights being around her ankles; laboratory tests were negative.

The remaining puzzle was that she had been strangled using a pair of tights wound four times around her neck, and a similar material had been used to bind her hands together. Surely it was odd that the person responsible must have had in his (or her) possession at the time two pairs of tights.

Most likely the assailant would have been someone she knew and had possibly arranged to meet, but not much more could be guessed. And there the matter rested, apart from the coroner's verdict of unlawful killing.

Some sixteen years later, however, more evidence came to light. A person contacted the police and told them that someone known to the girl and to the informant had committed the crime. The individual accused had been questioned closely at the time of the murder and been found to have a substantial alibi. Nevertheless, the new evidence was considered very seriously, and I had several interviews with detectives concerning its possible correlation with the original findings. Unfortunately, there had been no indication of any injury or blow to the head – nothing to indicate she had been incapacitated or concussed before being tied up, as was alleged by the informant.

Much as one would have liked to have the case reopened, the new evidence was flimsy at best and it was highly likely that, if it had reached court, the accused would simply have denied the allegation and, without forensic evidence, would have had to be discharged. Recent developments in DNA profiling, unavailable to us then, would have been a most useful tool, particularly as a number of laboratory exhibits and clothing from the deceased were still available. However, there were no further developments.

Unsolved murders involving teenage children increasingly hold the public's and the media's interest. Needless to say, there is often a sexual motive. Typically an unsuspecting youngster is sexually attacked when alone, or is apprehended while out on a walk and persuaded to accompany the criminal 'just for a walk'.

Not so in the case of a 13-year-old lad who left his home at Woodingdean, Brighton, in May 1967, for a stroll. His body was subsequently found on a bridle path in an area of the Sussex Downs known as Happy Valley, a well known picnic spot. The lad may have been killed in the pursuance of a robbery as the pockets of his trousers were turned inside-out and his pocket money, given to him by his father a mere hour before a passing girl came across the body, was missing.

It was thought that a vagrant – with possibly bloodstained clothing – could have been responsible. There was also a mysterious sighting of a shabbily dressed woman, about 40 years of age. Clad in a grey gaberdine raincoat, she was seen near the murder spot about the time that the body was discovered; she had also been noticed by several people earlier that day near a hall where a jumble sale took place in Ovingdean.

A rigorous search of the area for a murder weapon by the police and others was fruitless. Subsequently a possible murder weapon, a sharp single-edged serrated knife with a white bone handle, was discovered in the area. There was also a bloodstained seat on a Number 6 bus which would have stopped a few hundred yards from the bridle path – another possibly significant finding.

Did it all add up to a vicious assault by a female desperate for money who had acquired the knife from a local jumble sale that day and then escaped on a passing bus?

When I arrived at the scene shortly before midnight on the evening of his death, the boy lay adjacent to the bridle path, his chest on the thick grass of the verge of the path itself, in a semi-prone position. His clothing was undisturbed except for the trouser pockets. There was bloodstaining on his pullover and numerous tears through its thickness. A handkerchief lay on the grass nearby, plus a paper tissue closer to the body.

I found seven stab wounds on the front of the body, five of them on the neck, cheek and upper part of the chest and the remaining two penetrating the abdominal cavity. Additionally, there were six wounds on his back, some penetrating the lung. Numerous specimens were taken and retained for laboratory tests. Thirteen stab wounds, all of a similar nature, could only have been the result of, as they say in court, a frenzied attack, probably initiated from behind, with, as the boy lay on the ground, further grievous wounds being inflicted on his neck and chest.

On two occasions a few months later I examined the seven-inch-long knife which had been found. I had mentioned in my original report that there were distinctive pressure marks on the skin surface of some of the wounds, caused by an unusual projection at the base of the knife used. The knife I now examined did indeed have a distinctive pattern, as the base of the blade was separated from the handle by a loose metal collar, which was capable of movement. After comparing the knife with the wounds mentioned in my report and the photographs, I concluded there was no doubt that this weapon coincided with the shape and diameter of the wounds. The serrated edge of the blade could have accounted for the notched appearance of one edge of each wound. Pathologists are seldom dogmatic about the relationship between a murder weapon and wounds, but there was little room for doubt in this case.

Some thirty-five years have passed and no arrest has been made. A murder hunt is never officially put aside or forgotten by the police, and this tragic case has been the subject of review more than once over the passing years.

Chapter Thirteen

Dangerous Liaisons

As a matter of urgency I was called in July 1999 to a house in north London where a man, Patrick Willett, had been found dead on the sitting-room floor of his flat wearing only a pair of red pants. In the room I had limited means of manoeuvre, as it was quite small. The man's body was almost covered in blood, but some wounds were visible and they appeared to be of a stabbing nature.

While the body was taken to the mortuary for examination, I was informed about the victim's life. He was a single man, living alone, and I was not surprised when I was told he was suspected of homosexual liaisons. Blood tests for HIV are usually done routinely if such information comes to light, and autopsy precautions are taken to avoid coming into contact with the body other than through surgical gloves. Another hazard is hepatitis virus, tests for which are also routinely available. One can be overconscientious about taking care when carrying out a post-mortem, only to find that for some silly reason one nicks the surgical glove with a knife and first aid becomes essential. That nearly happened in this case. If the HIV test is reported as positive, one either makes a limited autopsy – not very satisfactory – or the autopsy is carried out in a specially equipped post-mortem theatre, of which there are few.

The man I examined was lying on his right side. Rigor mortis was established; he had probably been dead for some twenty-four hours before being found by a neighbour.

At my mortuary examination it was soon quite obvious externally that he was accustomed to homosexual acts. There were only a few small defence-type wounds on his left hand, made presumably as he had attempted to ward off his attacker; quite often there are a number of wounds of this nature. When I turned over the body I noticed a stabbing-type wound in the centre of his back, its margins sharply defined; it was only later that the significance of this wound would become apparent. My main attention was directed to a mass of stab wounds on the front of the body, eight on the side of his head, eight on the left side of the neck and ten on the left side of the chest, four of which had entered the deeper tissues, one passing through the heart into the liver – which was the wound that had caused his demise. There were also five superficial wounds on the top of the head. In all, then, amounting to thirty-two wounds.

I next examined the abdominal tissues and exposed the length of the spinal column, where I found the point of a knife protruding through the body of one of the main vertebrae, at the junction of the chest and abdomen. It was impossible to remove the knifepoint from the dense, hard spinal bone, so dissection of a single lumbar vertebral body was made. It was evident that the knife had passed right through the spinal cord, having reached there from the entrance wound I had seen on the deceased's back. It was just a matter of chance that I hadn't nicked the top of my finger on the sharp protruding edge as I was carrying out my abdominal examination.

Clearly, at the onset of the attack, a knife had been plunged straight through the man's back with enormous force while he'd been lying down. His assailant had pulled it out but in so doing had broken off the end of the blade.

Fresh appraisal of the wounds indicated that the man would

have been paralysed from the chest downwards as a result of that initial spinal stab, which had made it impossible for him to resist the onslaught of the other thirty or so blows rained upon his body. The knife responsible – missing its tip – was found in the flat's small kitchen.

I hadn't come across a case like this before; it was macabre. There followed police investigations by the CID for the man's homosexual associates, one of whom had seemingly entered the flat, probably with him, then stabbed him as described and finally set about him with a second knife.

It was not long before a man, John Barden, was arrested; blood samples from his clothing indicated his involvement with the death.

I was not required to attend the assize court at the Old Bailey, my evidence having been accepted by the defence team. Perhaps they thought that a detailed account of those dreadful wounds, particularly the stab through the back, would have made an unfavourable impression on judge and jury. Instead they simply described 'some thirty to thirty-five wounds'.

Subsequently I heard the exact circumstances of the case made available to the court. The deceased, Willett, the 34-year-old manager of a bingo hall, had met the accused, Barden, a 19-year-old soldier on leave in London, in a public house, and had offered him a room for the night at his flat. Once they got there, the soldier was put into the spare room and, while he was settling down for the night, his host appeared, wearing only his underpants, and began to pull back the bedclothes. Barden pulled out a knife he had placed under his pillow. Willett then left the room, returning with the kitchen knife and, in the words of the prosecution counsel, 'as if to do battle'. At this juncture Barden, out of fear for his life and under extreme provocation, attacked Willett. It is not clear where the second knife came from; it may have been the one held by the deceased, which the accused could easily have wrested off him following the initial back wound, although I had previously understood from detectives that the broken knife had been left on a draining board in the kitchen and a second carving knife had been taken from the cutlery drawer.

The soldier pleaded guilty to manslaughter and was acquitted of murder. He received an eight-year prison sentence. In his summing up the judge described the deceased as a 'seducer of stray boys'.

Occasionally a murder investigation is full of surprises, and so it was in the case of the death of George McKenzie. Initial assumptions were made which proved incorrect, and at the trial there was a remarkable volte-face in terms of the defendant's evidence.

A fire had broken out in a downstairs flat in a house in north London. Firemen called to the scene extinguished the blaze and found the body of a man, George McKenzie, lying fully dressed on the floor. A senior police surgeon attended the scene to certify death and give some guidance to police officers. He thought that the man had been overcome by fumes from the fire, and a very preliminary examination suggested that some form of electrical short circuit could have initiated the blaze. A short time later the CID arrived, and an astute woman detective constable drew her colleagues' attention to a discoloured towel wrapped across the man's neck. It had earlier been noticed by the fire crew, who thought nothing of it, but she regarded it as unusual and suspicious – and was proved entirely correct. When the towel was moved, a number of marks could be seen across the man's neck.

Owing to the disturbance of the room I did not attend the scene until I had completed the autopsy. The man was wearing a shirt, pullover and trousers, all intact except for a burn down the left trouser leg. His head hair was scorched. There was discoloration and blistering of the face and hands, and of the left leg. I noticed that the towel, which had already been removed from the neck when I saw it, was partially burnt. I heard that, owing to the necessity of extinguishing the fire, the room had been completely doused with many gallons of cold water, so I thought any estimate I gave for time of death would be unreliable. Quite rightly: although rigor was present, the body temperature was quite low, approaching room temperature, which would normally have indicated that he had died the previous day; it transpired that in fact his death had occurred just a few hours before the fire was noticed.

It was a complicated case to examine, as there were a number of highly significant marks on the front of the neck, a long graze across it with four separate ones on the right side of the neck, and a vertical one below the right jaw. This marking might have been caused by pressure exerted on the towel, but it was also possible that some of the marks might have been due to the deceased trying to release the towel. There were many asphyxial changes in the eyelids showing, without doubt, that he had struggled to breathe and had died through lack of air. However, there were more injuries beneath the surface of the skin of the neck – extensive bruising in the deeper tissues on the right side and a fracture of the cartilage of the voicebox, with internal bruising of the latter. There was no evidence of smoke being inhaled into the air passages, as would have occurred had he been alive at the time the fire started. This conclusion was confirmed by the complete absence of carbon monoxide in the bloodstream. In addition to signs of suffocation and/or strangulation associated with the towel on his neck, the internal bruising of the voicebox was due to a severe blow to the side of the neck, as pressure from the towel could not have caused the internal injuries.

More was to come, as there was also extensive bruising in the spaces between the lower ribs on both sides, chiefly the left, where two ribs were fractured. These injuries were due to heavy localized blows on both sides of the chest, more on the left, possibly caused by a right-handed man. It was beginning to look as if someone with a knowledge of boxing and/or karate could have been responsible for the man's injuries. This proved to be an important point in identifying the person who was eventually charged.

Subsequently Keith Mant came on behalf of the defence to discuss my findings and to see my final report. He agreed that pressure on the neck had been the cause of death, but I thought the blow on the neck could also have played a part. Obviously the fire was started in an attempt to cover up the crime – as is often the case, it was a singularly unsuccessful attempt.

Before the case was heard in the crown court – in this instance the Central Criminal Court at the Old Bailey – a hearing took place in the magistrates' court, basically to ascertain whether there was a case for the accused to answer concerning the prosecution's submission. Often enough this is a mere formality; very rarely is a case discharged at this level of legal process, and usually the pathologist is not called to give evidence.

I was called on this occasion, partly as the findings at autopsy were unusual; no doubt the defence wished to test the strength of the prosecution case concerning the cause of death. Defence counsel went into some detail regarding the significance of the blow to the neck. My view was that such a blow would cause obstruction to breathing and possibly interfere with those nervous impulses down the side of the neck that control the heart rate. While these views were accepted, the defence stated that the blows to his chest had been sustained in a sparring encounter the previous day. The deceased was engaged in teaching and supervising boys boxing at a club, a matter which became relevant as more information concerning his lifestyle was brought to light. However, I thought that the injuries could not have occurred twenty-four hours prior to his death, as in that case bruising would have been evident on the skin surface.

Reading my report of the committal proceedings, as they are called, I can see it was quite a long afternoon's work. The defence tried by various suggestions to limit the nature of the injuries to the man's neck, and muddy the waters as to which particular injury had caused death. As in the previous case, I was not called to give evidence at the Old Bailey. I had been told I would be required to attend the Central Criminal Court, but the trial terminated before I was required.

It was a 15-year-old schoolboy who was charged with killing McKenzie, who had been a local youth club worker. The boy pleaded not guilty to murder, manslaughter and arson. Michael Worsley QC, outlining the case for the prosecution, said the boy had strangled McKenzie with a towel after punching him. With the knowledge of the boy's parents, he had been allowed to spend the night at McKenzie's home; counsel emphasized there was nothing to suggest an improper relationship. Both the boy and McKenzie had been seen at 11 a.m. on the morning of the death. The latter's body was discovered shortly after 2 p.m., as an explosion was heard, caused by the crashing from the ceiling of plaster loosened by the intense heat from the fire.

Later that afternoon the boy had been seen by a friend and had said he'd been in a bit of trouble. While sparring with McKenzie he had accidentally punched him in the neck, whereupon McKenzie fell on the bed, went blue and looked dead.

The case was adjourned until the following day. Evidence was given that nothing was too much for McKenzie to do to help boys; he organized fishing trips, boxing, football and table tennis. But it was now revealed in court that there was a sinister side to his nature. His homosexuality had been fairly obvious to us from early on; what we had not known was that he had a perverted yen for youngsters. Defence counsel said that, since his arrest, the boy had been too ashamed to reveal the motive for the killing but had blurted it out to his parents after the first day of the trial. He said McKenzie had tried to assault him sexually, and in desperation to get away he had killed the man. The boy hated him 'for what he had tried to do to me. I had to stop him.' McKenzie had grabbed the boy and tried to kiss and fondle him. The boy had reacted out of panic, anger, disgust and fear. What had happened to McKenzie could in no way be justified, but it could be understood.

It transpired that the schoolboy, a boxing champion who completely trusted his mentor, become the target of McKenzie's lust. In a moment of blind panic the boy had killed him, and he was now prepared to plead guilty to manslaughter and arson.

The judge, James Miskin QC, cleared the lad of murder and placed him under the supervision of the Probation Service for two years. 'You are only fifteen,' he said. 'This occurred and you tried in vain to destroy the evidence. The Crown accepts the plea of manslaughter on grounds of provocation, as you had suffered a gross insult and completely lost control.' Miskin suggested that his previous denial was possibly a result of innate shyness.

It was revealed that McKenzie had been a member of several pornographic film clubs and had kept a diary in which he revealed homosexual activities. A neighbour had become suspicious of his activities, but not suspicious enough.

Many homosexuals are of course in stable relationships, but chance homosexual encounters may on occasion lead to blackmail threats, robbery, assault and murder. Such proved to be the case when I was called to Hampstead Heath, north London, where the partly decomposed body of a man, Malik Hattack, had been found. His death would result in the conviction of a violent robber, William Anderson – whose violence was all too evident at the autopsy. The deceased, a homosexual chauffeur, had been chatted up by Anderson in a west London pub and, presumably by mutual agreement, they had driven to a secluded spot on Hampstead

Heath. As well as being a renowned beauty spot, the heath has in recent years gained notoriety as a meeting place frequented by homosexuals, particularly after dark, often with persons quite unknown to each other participating in sexual acts.

However he was lured to the heath, the victim was subsequently found fully clothed, with his hands and feet bound by shoelaces. It was difficult to say whether the ties had been applied during life, because the heavy clothing he was wearing had obviated any marking of the skin of the feet or hands. I also found two socks coiled together impacted in the victim's mouth, and a ligature had been applied across the mouth and knotted on one side of the face. These restrictions alone had not necessarily caused his death and they, too, might have been applied after death, the cause of which was manual strangulation. There were massive asphyxial changes in the face and extensive bruising and trauma on both sides of the voicebox, caused by a deep compressive force exerted by thumb and fingers. The victim had been lying in the undergrowth for a day or so before discovery, fully clothed; apart from the trouser buttons being undone, there was nothing to suggest a sexual assault.

The arrested man, Anderson, was revealed as a most dangerous criminal who had been temporarily – and unwisely – released from the prison system. He had a host of convictions covering some ten years of violence and robbery; more recently, he had been jailed for five years. After serving two years of this sentence he was allowed weekend leave, without the requirement for a psychiatrist's report. The result was that within three days he had robbed a man in a London hotel – also leaving him bound hand and foot – and then, still on the loose, had encountered the chauffeur. After the attack he took his car and drove to Scotland, where he was tracked down and arrested.

Judge John Hazan imposed a life sentence with a recommendation that, in the interests of the public, Anderson should never be released until absolutely safe. Hazan also drew particular attention to the unfortunate circumstances surrounding Anderson's parole.

Daily papers often contain accounts of senseless assaults against and even the murders of young people taking a short cut on their way home late at night, having missed a bus or being unable to get a lift. Where girls are concerned, rape is often associated, and the girls may vanish until discovery of the body weeks later. On some occasions it appears that the perpetrator lies in wait, possibly habitually, for such chance encounters. Homosexual men run a much greater risk than heterosexual ones, as it is not unusual for such persons to be followed on their way to assignations.

The unfortunate homosexual – in fact, seemingly bisexual – man I have in mind chose on his way home from work to take a secluded pathway, which ran from a suburban road in north London, not to walk to his own home but for a relatively short detour (some 150 yards) into Highgate Woods. Highgate Woods, like Hampstead Heath, is noted for after-dark encounters between homosexuals.

The deceased was a married man in his forties, with a child; his habits were known to his wife and colleagues. He held an important post in the Home Office. On the night of his death he had been drinking with colleagues in a public house in Central London, and had then taken his usual underground train to travel home. It was not known whether he was alone. He was found the following morning lying fully dressed on the leafy verge of the pathway to the woods. His tinted spectacles lay nearby, and he had been robbed of his wallet, rings and watch; his tie was also missing. Police wondered whether he had been dumped there or if this was the actual scene of the crime. The fact that he was walking in the woods and not to his nearby home would seem to indicate his intentions, but on the other hand he had been waylaid, attacked and robbed with no signs of a sexual motive.

The investigation was coloured by two recent incidents in the same area. Almost a month previously a young man had been attacked in the nearby road, receiving a shattering blow to his skull, believed to be from an iron bar. A similar incident ten days earlier had involved another man being attacked with, it was thought, likewise an iron bar. Both attacks had fortunately not been fatal.

Obviously, by their nature, these previous attacks were relevant to the investigation, which made my findings more difficult to correlate. I knew the police thought the iron bar had been involved on this occasion too, but I found nothing to support that view. There was a distinctive injury to the victim's face, a black eye on the left side with considerable bruising of the tissues, and some skin grazing on his forehead. There was no injury to the underlying skull, as had occurred in the previous two cases, and, curiously enough, although there was no mark on his neck externally, there was massive damage to the underlying tissues, with bruising around the voicebox and fracture of the cartilage. Not unnaturally, there were also asphyxial changes resulting from the neck trauma.

I thought there must be an unusual explanation of these findings. It was obvious that he had been punched in the face initially, but there was no sign of active strangulation. He could have been mugged with a flexed arm applied to his neck by someone standing behind him, or he could have received a karate blow. Although by its very nature the latter is a blow delivered with the margin of the hand, in view of the previous attacks it was possible that a metal instrument, possibly that iron bar, had been swung against his neck – although I thought it highly unlikely in the absence of damage to his skull. The manner of his death was clear, but not the instrument which had caused it.

Unfortunately no one was ever apprehended. This tragic death was indirectly connected to the victim's homosexuality: there is little doubt that he was waylaid on his way to meet or seek a homosexual partner. He was just in the wrong place at the wrong time.

The finding of a man's body in a flat in Fulham in 1982 had unfortunate consequences for me, although the medical investigation was straightforward, if gruesome. It was a bizarre homosexual murder. He was last seen leaving a public house in Chelsea; his body was discovered when a fire alarm alerted neighbours. There were multiple stab wounds to the chest, but also incised mutilating wounds inflicted after death on the trunk and legs, and there was a ligature strangulation mark on the neck; a length of rope was found on the floor near the body. Furthermore, he had been castrated after death, the penis and scrotum being left on a nearby chair. Following the castration, a broken knife had been plunged into the groin wound.

It is customary for the pathologist to photograph the scene of a murder or, more particularly, the wounds. Although the officers of the Metropolitan Police photographic department take excellent full- and half-plate colour photographs nowadays for exhibit in court, these are sometimes not available for the pathologist to retain. Nevertheless, I had almost given up taking my own photographs as the police were so efficient. (Nowadays photographs taken by pathologists in connection with a case have to be made available to the court.)

I had completely forgotten photographing these gruesome scenes until an unpleasant incident occurred following the processing of the film. Some time later, I had taken on the same film a number of social and family photographs, and months later I gave it to my local chemist for processing. My wife called in once or twice to collect the prints, unsuccessfully, and we began to think it strange that the developing of our film was taking so long.

I became aware of the reason when a local detective sergeant called on me, bearing my photographs, which had been taken to the police station with the complaint that they depicted a sadistic orgy. The officer recognized me from my work as a pathologist as I had given evidence in a number of cases in his area, and so the matter, I thought, was closed at that point.

Not so. I received a hostile letter from the head office of the large pharmaceutical firm of which my local chemist was a branch. They expressed their entire dissatisfaction with the matter, and said they had given instructions to the branch chemist not to accept any further films for developing. I was so incensed by the letter that I consigned it forthwith to the dustbin.

I forgot all about the matter until, a while later, I went entirely innocently to the chemist with another film to be processed.

The manager looked at me and handed the film back with a gesture of distaste.

Chapter Fourteen

The Death of Ann Chapman

In the absence of ignorance and stupidity, Ann Chapman's futile and tragic death would not have occurred. It did so because she went to Greece at a sensitive time, during the military dictatorship that held power from 1967 until the return of democracy in 1974 with the government of Constantinos Karamanlis. Her own ignorance and the misinterpretation of her actions by agents of the Greek state, who judged her visit either important or sinister, led to her death. It was followed by years of seemingly fruitless efforts to see justice by her father, who was utterly determined to get at the truth and, at the same time, erase a slur on his daughter's character.

On 11 October 1971 Ann Chapman, aged 25, a journalist with a university background and an interest in Greek politics, left Gatwick among a party of sixteen colleagues for a ten-day visit to Corfu, Athens and the Greek islands, with the intention of publicizing Olympic Holiday Tours. She hoped to interview people out of favour with the government, and the evening before she disappeared had mentioned she had a big story in the offing.

On 14 October the party left Corfu, arriving at Pine Hills Hotel, Kavouri, half an hour north along the coast road from Athens. In the group was the Operations Manager of Olympic

Airways, Tellis Kotsias (who some years later would meet a mysterious death in a car that plunged into the River Thames at Walton, Surrey). The following day, 15 October, they went to Athens and, while most of the party toured the Acropolis, Ann stayed in the travel agency as she wished to contact various Greek tourist officials. She met the main group of journalists at 5 p.m. and thereafter all had free time until dinner, which had been arranged in an Athens hotel. Ann, in the company of another journalist, Nicholas Clarkson, returned to Pine Hills Hotel, while the remainder of the party stayed in Athens; she wished to change her clothing. The arrangement was that they would all meet in the Electra Hotel in Athens at 9 o'clock that evening. During the day – and there is nothing whatsoever to contradict this – Ann ate one sweet and drank a small amount of Ouzo for lunch.

Clarkson occupied an adjoining hotel room to Ann. He did not intend to return to Athens for dinner. He told Ann to catch the bus to Athens, the bus stop being 200–300 yards from the hotel. She left to catch the 7.45 p.m. bus, which would bring her into Athens sometime between 8.15 and 8.30 p.m. However, a taxi driver, Ionnis Phytos, stated in evidence that it was about that time that a girl from the hotel met outside it one of two men whom he had picked up previously from the local village.

Ann's absence from dinner was noted, and the following day the hotel manager went to her room to find that the bed had not been used and there was no sign of her. Her disappearance was reported to the police. Her body was found in a sheepfold near the bus stop on 18 October by a couple out looking for edible snails.

A detailed report by Captain Tsoutsias of the gendarmerie read:

The body was lying prone with the left cheek on the ground, almost covered with grass and thistles. Her hands were tied at the back with wire and the feet also tied. On the right cheek lay a large stone, some 70–80 kilo weight, one end propped against the ground, and a similar small stone, some 40 kilo, propped against the right elbow of the deceased, covering the forearm. The body was partly clothed and there were no trousers present and the pants showed some slight bloodstaining. There had been no attempt to remove the latter. The coloured blouse she wore was torn on the shoulder and her white brassiere had not been disturbed. There was no sign of a struggle in the vicinity or elsewhere and it had rained heavily over the weekend.

The state pathologist, Dr Demetrious Kapsaskis, arrived on the scene at 8 p.m. on 18 October, the evening her body was found, and he thought that death had probably occurred some forty-eight hours previously. He viewed the body at night with the aid of car lights, and then the following day carried out a detailed post-mortem examination.

He found that post-mortem hypostasis, which is due to simple gravitation of blood according to the position of the body, was on the front of the trunk and thighs, in keeping with the position in which she was found. Hypostasis was also present on the right shoulder, the upper part of the back and the right side of the chest. This unequivocally indicated that Ann's body had lain, immediately after her death, on her right side, the right shoulder and back against the ground and the left side upper-most. While the hypostatic change may occur within one to two hours of death, it is exceptional for it to remain visible if the body is moved during that time, as the initial hypostasis would tend to fade or gravitate elsewhere – in fact, it is usual to assume that some four to six hours elapse before hypostasis becomes 'fixed' in the tissues.

There were certain marks on the body due to its having been

dragged over rough ground: linear grazes on the backs of the lower thighs, the knee hollows and the upper calves, the upper margins being quite sharply defined. There was nothing on the feet or ankles.

The wire marks appeared to have been caused after death, as there was no sign of congestion or lividity at their margins and they were parchment-like in colour, the wire being knotted across the front of the legs and at the back of the hands.

Kapsaskis found some superficial injuries, bruising and grazing, including an injury to the left eye in keeping with a blow, and grazing and bruising of the breastbone, also in keeping with a blow with a fist or foot.

The more significant injuries were on the neck, where there was bruising around the strap muscles on each side of the voice-box. In particular, there was a mark on the skin of the right side of the neck, with underlying deep bruising and a fracture of the small bone which supports the voicebox. Kapsaskis also identified three lesser marks on the left side of the neck, in keeping with manual strangulation by a one-handed grip, caused by a right hand placed firmly across the front of the neck.

The only other finding was a small amount of food in the stomach, said to be of animal origin, consistent with it having been consumed an hour or two before death. It was thought to be the remains of a sandwich.

The pathologist's report included the critical feature of the case – that the body had been moved. It was concluded that the body had been moved less than seven hours after death and certainly not earlier than an hour and a half. The second pathologist present at the examination – as is customary under the continental system of autopsy – came to the conclusion that three to seven hours had elapsed before the body had been moved.

It seemed that the body had been held by the arms and feet by two people to be lifted and pulled along the ground to its place of concealment; if it had been dragged by one man, you would have expected to see grazing on the heels. Another explanation of the grazing elsewhere on the body would be that Ann had been pushed violently over the stone wall next to the bus stop, particularly if she had initially been sitting on it. There was, to repeat, no evidence of rape or sexual interference.

There had already been a series of searches in the vicinity of where her body was found. The day following the discovery of her body, a ring and driving licence were found near the wall of the sheepfold, and five days later her trousers were found under a stone some fifty yards away from where the body lay; a day later her handbag was discovered, with her sandals threaded through the handle. The fact that these articles, none discovered during the earlier search of the area, all came to light during further searches could possibly mean that someone placed them in position at various later times.

In summary, Ann had been attacked, punched in the face, knocked to the ground, strangled, tied, carried, dragged and partly hidden with two heavy stones on the body.

Her body returned to this country on 25 October. The Home Secretary had issued an order stating that neither an inquest nor a death certificate was necessary under the circumstances, and the go-ahead was given for cremation – normal practice at that time, but entirely different from procedures nowadays, when the coroner, if he or she has reasonable cause to suspect a violent or unnatural death within his or her jurisdiction, is obliged to conduct an inquest.

The Chapmans could not face identifying Ann's body. Still numb and in a state of shock, they asked a padre friend, the Reverend Eric Blennerhasset, a chaplain to Radio London who knew Ann, to identify the body for them. He agreed to do so, and reported back to Ann's father that he had noticed a parchment-like appearance of the face as she lay in the coffin.

Two years later, becoming increasingly suspicious about the

whole scenario, Mr Chapman checked on the possibility that his daughter's body had not in fact arrived in this country in that coffin, and he was astounded to hear from the undertakers that the seals on the casket had never been opened. This entirely contradicted Blennerhasset's account, and the matter was never satisfactorily resolved. The undertakers have, however, pointed out that they based their report that the coffin had never been opened on the fact that no charge had been made on the account for opening the casket, so it is possible the confusion was just a matter of clerical error.

Until August 1972 the following year, nothing much happened of interest. Edward Chapman, Ann's father, went to Greece, only to find himself being fobbed off by British Embassy and Consulate officials and given mere blandishments by the Greeks. However, two events occurred in August that year which altered matters. Mrs Chapman wrote a letter to the Greek authorities saying that she thought they knew Ann's killer. They did not, but coincidentally a Greek family row led to the arrest of a man who was later found guilty of Ann's murder.

This man was Nicolas Moundis, aged 34, who had surprised his wife ironing a pair of soldier's trousers, which was what had precipitated the row. He became violent, assaulting her, and is said to have exclaimed, 'I'll make you like Chapman.' His wife's aunt told a local policeman whom she knew, and within a short time Moundis had been arrested. He later alleged that he was told by the police that, if he cooperated, he would be paid a considerable sum of money and given a light prison sentence. He refused and was then the subject, according to him, of torture – in particular being dangled halfway out of a high window. After a mixture of threats and bribery, Moundis signed a confession which he subsequently retracted.

The story given in the confession was that he saw Ann at the bus stop and that she consented to go with him into a nearby field. All went well until Ann saw his wedding ring and he found she was menstruating. So we have a girl of impeccable character who speaks no Greek at all agreeing, with just a few minutes to spare before her bus arrives, to casual sex in a field with a complete stranger.

After being charged, Moundis was led on two arranged visits to the scene of the crime with the police, on 27 and 28 August. He said that no one left the car, but he was told how the girl had come out of the hotel to the bus stop and where the body was found. He was shown the wire and also the scenes where the handbag and trousers had been found. Later, on 31 August, he was again taken there, and an official reconstruction was arranged with an attorney and pathologist present, Moundis being reminded beforehand of how he had climbed the wall and precisely where the two lovers had lain on the ground. By this time he had been charged with murder. The reconstruction was well publicized, and by chance the serial photographs taken during it came into my hands, via Mr Chapman. The reconstruction seen in the photographs showed quite clearly Moundis demonstrating how he had suffocated the deceased. In fact, she was strangled.

On 3 April 1973 Moundis was tried, his defence depending on an alibi which related to a matter on which he had earlier been questioned. He was, in fact, in Kavouri that evening, having gone there to meet a girl he had propositioned the day before in Athens. She didn't appear and so he looked around, spying on courting couples, one of his favourite pastimes. Later he went home, being picked up by a taxi driver who, by sheer chance, was his uncle, the time being 10–10.30 at night. So if Moundis had killed Ann he would have had to have done so around 8.15 p.m., tied up the body and scattered her possessions at random, and then left the scene in time to be in Athens two hours after the initial attack. There are obviously glaring anomalies in this scenario – for one, the pathologist had said that Ann's body was moved three to seven hours after death.

Nicholas Clarkson, the last to see her, and the snail seekers were not called to give evidence at the trial.

It is highly unlikely that Moundis had anything to do with Ann's death for the following reasons. The time of death, although imprecise, would not have allowed sufficient time for him to commit the murder and return to Athens when he did so. As mentioned, there was no sign of sexual interference or rape, and the reconstruction indicated the wrong mode of death – Moundis obviously did not know how she had died. He was left-handed, but the strangulation marks on Ann's neck were typical of those caused by a right-handed person (unless, of course, she had been attacked from behind). There was also the unexplained food in the stomach. It is difficult to assess the significance of this, as it appeared that, although she hadn't eaten for many hours on the day of her death, she had nevertheless taken food several hours before the murder – a conundrum.

Ann's father thought the trial had been rigged. His lawyer believed that Ann might have been a small-time courier who had caused embarrassment to the military regime, and that Moundis would be quietly released. Chapman exerted pressure on the authorities; of course, the fall of the Greek junta in 1974 gave him added impetus. It was about this time that he came to me and, having read the evidence available, I came to the conclusion that Moundis was innocent of the charge of murder.

I went to Athens in May 1976 to give evidence to the Public Prosecutor and was required to express my views both to him and to the state pathologist, Dr Kapsaskis. For an unusual reason – he was recovering from a recent eye operation – the confrontation took place in the pathologist's flat in the presence of his wife, who interrupted proceedings from time to time. This was, needless to say, most irregular. Our discussion took most of the day, lengthened by the fact that everything had to be translated from English to Greek and back to English, although I subsequently discovered that Dr Kapsaskis understood and spoke English fluently. I pointed out that, although the findings of the medical investigation were correct, there were grave discrepancies in interpretation and conclusion.

The appeal that Moundis lodged with the Greek Supreme Court failed due to lack of new evidence, and in 1980, after a new (socialist) government had come into power, a second appeal was also defeated.

All seemed lost until 1982, when Richard Cottrell, then the Chapmans' Euro MP, told Chapman of his right as an EEC citizen to petition the European Parliament for redress of a grievance against an authority in another member state of the European Community. A petition was presented on Mr Chapman's behalf by Mr Cottrell.

There was an explosive atmosphere in the committee that heard the matter when a Greek deputy supported the petition, on the grounds that Ann's murder was the result of a political conspiracy. The petition in 1984 to the European Parliament voted to support it on the ground that Ann Chapman had been a victim of agents of the military regime. A few months later Moundis was released by a presidential edict, although he has never been pardoned. It was clear that the interpretation and significance of the medical findings had been tailored to suit the Greek authorities.

The Chapman case had received a great deal of publicity in Athens, particularly in the newspapers, and my arrival at the airport and my meeting with the prosecutor brought further attention to it. I should have realized that my presence would cause embarrassment to some in authority; so it was that, one evening after dinner, I had a call from the hotel lobby to meet a man who had asked to see me. He told me that he was there on behalf of Mr Chapman, who had arranged a small celebration. We walked some distance to a small street off the main thoroughfare, and down some steps to a small club of sorts. There was no evidence of Chapman. I was offered some drink. I gained the impression that my hosts were not sure of the purpose of my visit to Athens as they asked about the case of the dead journalist. More drinks followed, then a request to pay for the hospitality – which seemed quite exorbitant. I signed my American Express cheques as payment and these were accepted, confirmation of the men's ignorance of their use.

I decided to leave before matters became unpleasant, and persuaded the man who had brought me to return with me to the hotel on the pretext that I would show him some important documents and settle the rest of the bill. As I walked there with him I watched him carefully. We reached the hotel and he tried to grab me. I kicked out, then dived through the door – much to the surprise of the concierge, who helped me upstairs. I stayed in bed recovering for most of the next day, managing to tele-phone my bank in London to cancel all cheques. Later I met Chapman at an interview. He was quite shocked by my story.

In 1978 the owner of an art gallery in central Athens claimed he had seen Ann alive at his shop at the time she was supposed to be dead. His view and evidence were highly circumstantial, but six months later his home was burnt to the ground and he within it. In March 1983 the respected editor of a Greek news-paper, who had vigorously reported Chapman's efforts, was assassinated in his office. And during the course of his inquiries in Athens, Cottrell had been warned off the case. I feel that I had a lucky escape.

Chapter Fifteen

Foreign Affairs

A British pathologist may be called upon to investigate a death overseas, either on behalf of a person being held in custody on account of a suspicious death or murder or for an organization such as Amnesty International.

Occasionally, very occasionally, a post-mortem examination reveals a cause of death entirely contrary to that previously accepted. Such was the case at Uxbridge, Middlesex, one morning in March 1976, when in the presence of two senior detectives I examined the body of a ship's carpenter, aged 35, flown back to this country after being found dead in his cabin on a cargo ship which was at anchor in the Persian Gulf, off Kuwait City. The police officers had recently returned from Kuwait where a merchant seaman in the ship had been charged with the murder.

There had been considerable friction between the two seamen throughout the voyage concerning the amount of alcohol available to the ship's company, for which the deceased had been responsible. It culminated in a brawl, after which the deceased had retired to his cabin, where he was found dead the following day. It was thought he had sustained a serious injury during the altercation, and a Kuwaiti pathologist found he had died from a traumatic rupture of the spleen. The spleen lies just beneath the ribs in the upper abdominal cavity, and a blow in that area may cause rupture, particularly if it is already diseased.

I was surprised, perhaps less so than the detectives present, when at my examination I found no evidence at all of rupture of the spleen; the abdominal cavity was full of fluid due to advanced cirrhosis of the liver, but the spleen was intact. It appeared to have been wrenched from its attachment (pedicle) during the initial autopsy, there being no haemorrhage or bruising in the abdomen or around or in the spleen. It was clear that the man's death had had nothing to do with an affray and drastic action was necessary as the accused was facing trial for manslaughter in Kuwait the following week.

Within a few days I was requested, on behalf of the Department of Trade and Industry, to be their representative at the trial. I arrived in Kuwait in time for the court hearing, which was conducted before three trial judges – the prisoner, along with others, being visible behind the iron bars of the court. I anticipated difficulty and possible hostility in explaining the true state of affairs, and a consequent miscarriage of justice. After outlining my findings, I emphasized there was not the slightest evidence of violence having caused the man's death, and I presented to the court a specimen of a spleen which had been ruptured following a traumatic impact.

Sometimes such a rupture does not occur immediately. Instead a blow splits the substance of the organ, allowing blood to accumulate under the lining (capsule) until, after a day or even longer, the organ ruptures into the body cavity. Nothing of that nature had occurred here, as there had been no blow to the area of the man's spleen. His death was due to liver failure following cirrhosis of the liver, the most likely cause being chronic alcoholism. The specimen had the required effect on the court and, after a short discussion, the judges dismissed the case and ordered the man's release.

Subsequently I gathered the sailor had been taken back to the jail, given his possessions and released to fend for himself. I also discovered that any fee that I might submit would have to be recompensed by the accused from his pay. It was not a situation conducive to my claiming a substantial sum.

The Kuwaiti barrister was highly delighted. Previously he had confided to me that there was little chance of an acquittal. He took me to his limousine and drove me to his mansion, where he invited me to his study to discuss the case and partake of refreshment. He proudly showed me his 'books', which occupied three walls of the room. In fact each 'bound volume' concealed a bottle of alcohol – aperitif, brandy, liqueur or malt whisky. Surprising, as Kuwait is supposedly a dry country. On the remaining wall there was an illuminated full-length picture of a nude model.

I gathered the Kuwaitis were happy that the case had been settled.

Physicians for Human Rights, founded some twelve years ago, is a US-based non-profit organization whose goal is to bring the skills of medicine and science to the protection of human rights. It is voluntarily aided. Pathologists as well as clinicians from the USA and other countries may be called upon, often at short notice, to assist in the investigation of a possible torture or death in custody.

In November 1990, on their behalf, I flew to Israel to check on the death of a Palestinian prisoner, aged 32, who had been held in the Gaza military prison. He was taken into custody on 20 October, visited some nine days later by his family, and found hanging in his cell on 2 November. A detailed examination of his clothes and of his body showed no signs of assault.

There were characteristic marks caused by self-suspension. There were no signs of strangulation or physical violence, or of restraint by another person, and no evidence of a karate blow to the neck. There was nothing, in short, to suggest foul play. In addition, there were no signs of accidental hanging.

I carried out my examination in the presence of an old friend and colleague, Dr Yahuda Hiss, who had spent some months in the department at Charing Cross Hospital in 1985 and become the senior pathologist at L. Greenberg Institute of Forensic Medicine.

It was important that I visited the cell where the deceased had been found, to check whether it was possible for him to suspend himself – a vital part of the investigation – and take into account the dimensions of the cell; also to talk to staff and, finally, to examine the piece of blanket he had used to suspend himself.

As a result of these investigations, I concluded that it would not have been feasible for any person to cause the man's death by foul play and then simulate hanging by suspending his body afterwards. In my report I pointed out that, for suicide, it was not only necessary for death to occur by hanging but that the deceased should appreciate the likely result of his actions and that the balance of his mind was not disturbed.

In dealing with the organization for which I had voluntarily appeared I had to answer every possible question that might be raised by the family lawyer on behalf of the Palestinian Liberation Organization, who, in such situations, sometimes find difficulty in accepting explanations which do not fit their original ideas. I gained the impression that they did, indeed, suspect that the prisoner had been murdered in some way. They expected me to find in their favour, but of course I could not. A letter to me from Jonathan Fine, the Executive Director of Physicians for Human Rights, emphasized the importance of the organization in building trust in all parties concerned in forensic consultations, and the importance, too, of an independent inquiry. He complimented me on my mission, which was regarded as highly satisfactory.

Although pathologists find, from teaching and experience, that homicidal hanging is highly unlikely, it is important to keep the possibility in mind. The deaths of Roberto Calvi and possibly Rudolf Hess leave room for debate, so a pathologist should not automatically exclude homicidal hanging.

A case in Malaysia in 1987 provided such an opportunity. It involved the death of the son of a wealthy millionaire. The son had been found hanging in his bedroom. The matter was investigated at an inquest; although I had expected to attend, I was not required as my opinion was accepted by the court.

The deceased had been found in his luxurious house by his brother-in-law. Entry to the house was difficult, owing to the nature of the building and its security devices, but eventually access was gained to the room where the body was found via a hole in the wall left where an air-conditioning plant had been taken out temporarily for repair.

The man was found, wearing pyjamas, lying in the middle of the room near his bed. His hands were tied in front of his body. There was a massive ligature around his neck, consisting of plastic telephone cable wound round nine times with two free ends and five knots in front of the neck. A wire coat hanger encircled his left wrist, then passed in front of his left thigh, behind his right thigh and around his right wrist. The apparent point of suspension for this extraordinary multiple ligature contraption was from a hook in the ceiling immediately above the deceased.

The pathologist who carried out the autopsy found the cord on the deceased's neck was made up of two pieces, one wound six times and the other three times round the neck. More unusually, there was partial separation of two vertebrae in the uppermost part of his spine. From the appearances, it was obvious this was not a suicidal hanging in the usual sense of the term. A moderate amount of alcohol was found in the man's body, equivalent to five or six single measures of whisky, which he had taken the previous evening in the company of his brother-in-law. Presumably the hanging took place before 1 a.m., as the lights in the house were extinguished at that hour.

Many tests were carried out on the tensile strength of a similar cable, and these indicated that the ligature had originally been in one piece but that it had broken during the process of hanging. Though the officer who attempted to reconstruct the case said the hanging could possibly have been carried out by the deceased – that is, he could have put the cord round his own neck, tied his own wrists together and manoeuvred a loop over the hook in the ceiling – when the details were considered it was reckoned virtually impossible for him to have carried out the complicated manoeuvre with the wire coat hanger and suspend himself. We tried to reconstruct the scenario in the department – my colleagues being somewhat apprehensive of the idea which, of course, did not involve using as complicated a ligature – and we came to the same conclusion. There were some quizzical looks and wry expressions from my colleagues, who probably thought it was just another of the Prof's harebrained ideas.

In retrospect, after drinking whisky, the deceased, unaided, would have had to stand in the middle of the room on a stool 32 in high, supporting a cable 14 ft in length, and stretched upwards. As he was 5 ft 7 in tall, he had to stretch a further 26 in to reach the hook in the ceiling and place the cable over it. It would have been necessary to stretch his arm to its full extent, bring the cable down, loop it nine times round his neck and tie it five times in front of his neck; moreover, he would have had to put the coat hanger wire around his wrists after passing it between his legs and, finally, kick away the stool to suspend his body and cause his own death.

Tensile-strength tests of the cord confirmed that his fall would have caused it to break, so that he landed on the ground in a kneeling position with his head lying between the legs of the stool.

As far as we knew there was no motive for him to take his life, and the damage to the spinal column bone could equally have been caused by a blow across the neck as following suspension.

The death was highly suspicious and the circumstances suggestive of murder. The brother-in-law, who had found him, was arrested but later released. Subsequently the brother-in-law's solicitors wrote to the deceased's father informing him that there had been a conspiracy between several persons in order to make the deceased's suicide appear to be a murder. At the coroner's court, where proceedings had been adjourned on a number of occasions, the pathologist who carried out the autopsy finally agreed that the victim had been murdered in a strangulation-simulating hanging, and the coroner returned a verdict of homicide against person or persons unknown. The death remains a mystery.

Chapter Sixteen

Crash Landings

Flying, while usually a relaxing way to travel and providing enormous benefits generally, may occasionally result in a disaster – due to mechanical failure of the aircraft, human error or human miscalculation. The three aircraft disasters with which I have been concerned covered all three of these aspects. Two of the disasters occurred at a major airport, London Heathrow – one of these in broad daylight with no weather problems and witnessed by a number of people, including one with a cine camera. There is, of course, a 'black box' usually available following an aircraft disaster, which concerns matters of the aircraft's flight, so the pathological investigation is normally associated rather with identification of the dead and discovering the presence of natural disease, drugs and injuries.

On a Friday evening, 30 November 1975, I was anticipating a relaxing weekend when a call came from a coroner's officer to stand by as a light aircraft had been reported to have crashed on Arkley Golf Course, some five miles from where I live. Graham Hill, the World Motor Racing Champion in 1962 and 1968, had been piloting his twin-engine six-seater Piper Aztec back from Spain with his team after testing a racing car for the forthcoming season. He had retired from active racing the previous year, having taken part in 176 Grand Prix races, and was intent on developing his own team. His passengers included Tony Brise, his protégé, who had been showing great promise on the Grand Prix scene, as well as two mechanics, his manager and an engineer – six people in all. They had apparently decided to return earlier than originally planned in order to attend a function for Grand Prix drivers the next day. The plane's destination was the Elstree private aerodrome, some three or four miles from the site of the crash and quite close to Hill's home at Shenley. His expected time of arrival, confirmed by the control office at Elstree, had been 9.30 p.m., but unfortunately the weather conditions were poor – a typical English November evening with freezing fog and mist.

Tragedy struck. As the aircraft lost altitude on its flight path over Barnet, it brushed the tops of some trees and, destabilized, hit the ground. It disintegrated on impact and exploded as it went into a copse. There were no survivors.

In such an incident, once the crash is confirmed, the coroner is informed and, apart from calling the pathologist – in this case myself – he or she assembles a backup team, with a dentist and others necessary for photography and collection of specimens, together with Department of Transport officials and possibly another pathologist, from the RAF Institute.

Speed is of the essence, and in this case the coroner, Dr David Paul, was on hand to help overcome any administrative snags that might arise. Obviously the main purpose was to identify the victims and their injuries in relation to the plane's impact; also to try to ascertain if natural disease or collapse of the pilot might have been involved, or any other factors such as carbon-monoxide poisoning from a faulty heater. Toxicology is done as a matter of routine.

The crash and impact on the ground resulted in fatal injuries to all six persons in the aircraft, identification being complicated by the explosion, which caused extensive burns after death. Dental examination and referral to past records became vitally important. Bernard Sims, the forensic odontologist, framed his report in each case in the following terse manner:

Dental examination and identification carried out on the plane's occupants, based on the dental records and radiographs submitted by the dental surgeon, when related to the fatalities and compared with the autopsy charting, indicated eighteen points of reference in each instance, confirming identity.

No other form of identification was possible.

A few years earlier Graham Hill had sustained very severe injuries while racing, but there was nothing to indicate the resultant leg fractures were relevant or causing him any trouble at all at the time of the crash, and clearly he was a healthy and robust man, only 46 years of age.

Once the medical findings had been concluded, the report on the crash was passed to the Accident Investigation Authority, who compiled a report. There was no evidence of mechanical failure of the aircraft or incapacity of the pilot. While there was nothing specifically to explain the crash, it appeared that the pilot had been mistaken as to his distance from the airfield, and thus had descended prematurely. He was, we should remember, attempting to land in poor visibility at an airfield without appropriate landing aids.

Apart from the tragedy itself, which had devastating effects on the family, there were also matters relating to the validity of insurance, and these led to litigation on behalf of the other victims.

An entirely different form of aircraft disaster occurred on 27 October 1965, this time involving a turbo-prop BEA Vanguard aircraft. The density of traffic at London Heathrow is well known, involving millions of take-offs and landings each year, but fortunately there have been very few fatal plane accidents at the airport in the past forty years.

Again bad weather was a crucial factor. The plane from Edinburgh, with thirty passengers and six crew, had encountered thick fog as it approached London. It had been held for an hour by Air Traffic Control; visibility at the time varied, according to observers, between 110 and 600 yards. After making two initial approaches to land, the plane crashed on the runway, some halfway along, and burst into flames. There were no survivors.

The report of the public inquiry as to the reason for the accident – a document of some fifty pages – made it clear that there was no single cause. There were a number of complications related to landing, associated with problems of overshooting the runway, procedures associated with choice of movement of flaps, and the use of instruments.

At Uxbridge I was one of a team of three pathologists assembled to deal with the identification of the deceased by examination of clothing, valuables, documents and dental records. We worked throughout the night on this grim task with little respite, but were fortunate to have a well organized mortuary with all facilities instead of, as sometimes occurs, having to make do with makeshift accommodation and personnel.

A plane flying at its normal speed for landing sustains massive deceleration when it hits an immovable object, in this case the runway, as the forward movement is rapidly eliminated. Apart from the disintegration of the structure being likely to cause severe injuries to the passenger, the force of the impact is transmitted to the passenger's body and internal organs. The most susceptible internal area in such circumstances is the main vessel from the heart, specifically the point where the main blood vessel, the aorta, leaves the heart and curves around the centre of the chest to travel down the body. Deceleration forces can snap the vessel in two, producing a catastrophic haemorrhage and virtually instantaneous death.

In the 1965 Heathrow disaster almost every passenger died from this type of tear of the aorta. It may be of some comfort to grieving relatives that the end came very swiftly: there was certainly no time for cognisance of impending doom.

Is there any possibility of preventing such an event occurring? If any skeletal injuries are survivable and there is no fire on board, it might be possible. Some years ago Donald Teare suggested that passenger seats should be placed so that they faced the rear of the aircraft, thus eliminating sudden traumatic strain of this nature. The theory was sound, but the idea was not explored as the cost of reversing all aircraft seats would be monumental. And would the passengers *feel* safer facing the tail of the aircraft, particularly if the reason were explained?

Another disaster, quite unique in this country, occurred at Heathrow Airport on 3 July 1969. It was a bright warm summer afternoon when an Air Speed Ambassador twin-engine aircraft belonging to an independent airline prepared to land following a flight from Deauville, France. This was a commercial plane used for transporting horses, and it was bringing eight very valuable brood mares to stud farms in southeast England. Including the pilot and his colleague, there were twelve people aboard. As the plane descended to the runway, it struck two parked BEA aircraft, ended up against the ground floor of the terminal building, and rolled over on to its back. It had narrowly missed one Trident-type aircraft, with fifty passengers aboard, which was about to take off, sliced through the body of a parked Trident, and took the tail off another one, doing damage estimated at five million pounds – not taking into account the deaths of six on board the aircraft. Six passengers survived with injuries, and twenty-nine people on the ground were injured.

How did this bizarre accident occur? Following the task of identifying the bodies, the examination concentrated on any abnormality of the cardiovascular system of the crew and on routine toxicology tests, all of which showed negative findings. Another possible factor – quickly eliminated – was that the horses might have panicked on landing and broken loose from their stalls, upsetting the equilibrium and balance of the plane.

The answer to the question finally came from the investigation team, which showed that a failure of the port flap operating rod, due to metal fatigue, had caused the port flap to retract. The starboard flap extended further, leading to a rolling movement to port that became uncontrollable. An attempt to overshoot was impossible owing to the aircraft becoming increasingly difficult to control.

The report also drew attention to the post-mortem examination of the grooms, whose injuries indicated that they had been thrown about in the aircraft. This led to the suggestion that some form of safety harness would be useful in such circumstances, when the grooms would be standing by their charges ready for landing.

Forensic pathology has always been concerned indirectly with pointing the way to a better understanding of conditions and factors which cause death. The hazards of flying are no exception.

The last ten years have seen an increasing awareness of danger to passengers on long-haul flights and, in the last year before the time of writing, reports in the medical press and media have been increasingly concerned with a condition dubbed Economy Class Syndrome, initially described by two doctors and reported in a medical journal in 1977. The article referred to the potentially fatal condition of pulmonary embolism, which results when a blood clot breaks away from a thrombus in the leg vein, formed as a result of prolonged sitting. This condition can occur in passengers on long-haul flights. However, as early as 1940 Keith Simpson[1] found that a number

[1]Simpson, K., 1940, *Death from pulmonary embolism*, Lancet, **2**, 744.

of deaths in air raid shelters during the London Blitz were caused by pulmonary embolism. At that time London Underground station platforms were crowded by those seeking shelter and a safe place during the night. With official permission, they bedded down, some using garden deck-chairs. It was noticed that people on occasion collapsed and died as they left the shelters. The cause, Simpson pointed out, was pressure and constriction of the veins at the back of the knees, causing clotting of the bloodstream and leading to release of clots into the circulation, blocking the heart, the last link in this chain occurring as they left their sitting position.

Decades later, as a pathologist working in west London, near London Heathrow, I too became aware of such occurrences. The typical story is of a middle-aged woman who complains of feeling faint following a long-haul flight and then collapses on the airport concourse. Initially the fatalities were suspected to be due to heart attacks, but post-mortems showed the typical features of a pulmonary embolism. My colleague Dr R. Sarvesvaran[2] wrote a valuable survey of some four years' work during which a quarter of the airport deaths referred to the coroner were due to pulmonary embolic blood clots, almost all in females.

These observations and other papers did not cause much interest at the time; but more recent media coverage has emphasized the need for passengers to move about as much as possible during flight – not an easy thing to do – and, more practicably, to exercise the leg muscles on long-haul flights. Recent reports suggest that one in ten of all such passengers may develop a blood clot, leading to a figure of some 1,000 deaths throughout the world annually. A study by the World Health Organization, which will take two and a half years, has not yet commenced

[2]Sarvesvaran, R., 1986, *Sudden natural death associated with commercial air travel*, Med. Sci & Law, **26**, (1), 35.

through lack of funds. Although Britain has contributed substantial finances to the investigation, other governments have refused to help.

So there are other causes of air-travel death apart from trauma. Passengers have a statistically greater chance of dying through sitting immobile during a long flight than they have of ever being involved in an aircraft crash.

Chapter Seventeen

Electrocution

Homicidal electrocution is, by all accounts, exceptionally uncommon. The old chestnut bandied about by undertakers and morticians – and, dare I say it, on occasion by pathologists – is 'A Shocking Business'.

Successful murder by electrocution is difficult in that opportunity and means seldom coincide. From the pathologist's viewpoint, too, electrocution murders are problematic: if a death has occurred in a domestic environment, the possibility of deliberate electrocution having been the cause may be overlooked and the electrocution marks are often very inconspicuous and easily missed.

Let us look at some examples. A 39-year-old woman, Inkevi Collins collapsed in September 1959 at work at a north London factory. There was no obvious cause of death but, when I examined the body in some detail, I found there were two small brownish indentation marks on one finger. No doubt about it – these were marks of contact between the skin and an electric current, although I had never before seen a case. Her employers were unhelpful, but it transpired that her job involved assembling Christmas-tree lights, putting on the tiny lampshades and testing the bulbs. We found that the particular item she was examining at the time of her collapse included a plastic-covered wire; at one point the plastic covering had worn away so that the wire made contact with her hand, electrocuting her. Some years later her husband was awarded substantial damages in the High Court against the firm.

A not-dissimilar case with regard to an electric mark, although the circumstances were entirely different, occurred when a small boy collapsed and died as he ran through his parent's kitchen on a hot, humid summer afternoon. The doctor thought the 5-year-old could have died of epilepsy, as there had been convulsions after the collapse. The death was reported to the coroner. At examination I found pinpoint marks on the undersurfaces of the thumb and the first finger of the right hand. These marks were clearly those of electrocution, although the parents denied the possibility. Further investigation and tests by the electricity authority confirmed the truth.

As the lad had run through the narrow kitchen he had stumbled against and fallen on to an old cylindrical vacuum cleaner that was plugged into an electric socket in the wall. Although the switch was in the 'off' position, the terminal lead in the plug was incorrectly placed and the motor within the cylinder casing was not secure. When the child fell after tripping over the cleaner, the motor moved and came into contact with the metal casing, rendering it 'live' and causing a lethal shock to his finger. The parents were sceptical and deeply distressed, and it required a long explanation at the coroner's court before they could accept the verdict.

Occasionally an electric current is used as an adjunct to sexual stimulation. One young man wound a length of exposed metal wire around both lower forearms, connected through a resistance to an on-off switch. He apparently gained satisfaction by very rapidly using the push-through switch to give himself an evanescent shock. Unfortunately, his reaction time on one occasion was too slow, and he died immediately from electrocution as the current entered his body.

Attempted homicidal electrocution is not unknown, a case in point being one mentioned by Francis Camps in his forensic textbook, *Practical Forensic Medicine* (with W.B. Purchase). It concerned an ingenious apparatus set up by a man intent on giving his wife a fatal electric shock as she took a bath (R. *v.* Whybrow, 1952). He attached a wire to the metal soap dish in the bathroom and then ran it through the wall to a two-pin socket secreted in a cupboard. This was connected to a 15 watt bulb and switch, thence to a flex and a 15 amp wall plug. It is curious that he thought it necessary to introduce the lamp, because doing so only decreased the electric shock sustained by his wife when she touched the soap dish while taking her bath. The shock was further reduced because she was well insulated in the bath, the waste plug being in place. Perhaps he intended to give his wife only a nasty shock; in any event he was charged with attempted murder and received a custodial sentence.

More sinister was a simulated accidental electrocution perpetrated in a maisonette in Hayes in 1968. An Asian woman, Jean Northover, aged 30, was found lying in night attire on her back on the floor of the kitchen, her head inside the larder cupboard. She had a small domestic knife between the first and second fingers of her right hand. The cupboard contained a bank of wooden fuseboxes – old-fashioned by present-day standards. Some of the fuses were missing, having been removed from their sockets. Specifically, two fuses lay on the floor between her legs, one near her right leg, and two on the floor inside the cupboard. The appearance was that of a person receiving an electric shock while attempting to repair a defunct fuse. There were pathological signs to support this view: a number of quite characteristic electrocution marks were present on and between the fingers of both hands.

More detailed examination, however, showed signs of asphyxia in the eyelids and on the surface of the eyes. A form of asphyxia is not, curiously enough, an uncommon mode of death in electrocution: there may be spasm and contraction of the chest wall and the muscles between the ribs, restricting the victim's breathing. Here the asphyxial signs were associated with a number of superficial injuries on the face, in the form of tiny crescentic grazes and marks around the mouth – consistent with asphyxia caused not by electric current but by the presence of a hand against the mouth; suffocation, in other words.

In view of the electrocution marks, an electrical engineer carried out an inspection of the maisonette. The true state of affairs surrounding Jean Northover's death came to light when police interviewed the couple who occupied the upstairs maisonette. Their electric light and power were controlled by the fuseboxes downstairs. While they had been watching television that evening, the lights and power in the maisonette had temporarily failed. When the neighbours went downstairs they saw a man who pleaded with them to keep quiet about his presence in the maisonette.

Naturally they now informed the police of this. Later, when the man – Mrs Northover's husband – was arrested, he denied any knowledge of the matter. His alibi was that he had been on night shift at the nearby factory. Certainly no one had noticed his absence.

The prosecution case was that he had slipped away from work and entered the house. He had sufficient knowledge of electricity to have, in happier times, installed the electric circuit. After an argument and a struggle with his wife, he placed his hand over her mouth, causing her to lose consciousness; as he was wearing soft woollen gloves, any marks on her neck or face were minimal. He then arranged an electric wire around her hands and between her fingers as she lay in the pantry, plugging the other end of the wire into a 13 amp socket, taking out the fuses to simulate an accident. It was impossible to say if she had died directly from the effects of the electricity, the official cause of death being given as asphyxia associated with an attempt at electrocution.

The husband admitted in court that he had visited his wife. His counsel maintained that she had died unexpectedly following an argument sparked off by her grave provocation. The accused had placed his hand over her face to prevent her screaming or shouting and then, when she lost consciousness, had attempted in panic to mask his actions by rigging up the electrical apparatus and placing the small knife in her hand. This theory was not sustainable in court, as the asphyxial changes present indicated a significant degree of pressure across the mouth.

He pleaded guilty to manslaughter and was sentenced to six years' imprisonment.

As noted, electrical marks can be easily missed despite detailed examination of the deceased. This was true in a case of a lad of five who was found dead beside the electrified railway track at the sidings of Edgware, north London, after the motorman in the cab of a train had heard a cry from the track.

The lad had left home one afternoon at 4 p.m. on his BMX bike, dressed in a polo-neck jumper, shirt and cotton trousers. When he was found he was completely naked. His body was generally dusty and dirt-stained, with multiple grazes and scratch marks scattered irregularly over it, more on the back than the front. These were all superficial, both broad and fine in nature. It certainly appeared that he had run through some sort of thorny undergrowth.

My examination of the superficial external injuries presented a very extensive picture. The boy's hands were dirt-ingrained but initially seemed free of injuries. Two days later, however, I received a call from the mortician mentioning a peculiar mark on one hand. I went to the mortuary, and found a characteristic tiny electrical mark on the palm surface of the left hand. Such an injury, rather like a bruise, may become more evident or more prominent over the course of a few days.

The boy's death had been a consequence of his abduction by a 20-year-old neighbour, who had taken him to wasteland, stripped him of his clothing and indecently assaulted him. The terrified boy managed to escape the clutches of his attacker, running through the undergrowth down the embankment for some 150 yards towards the electrified railway line and his death. Whether he came into direct contact with electricity or whether a high-voltage flash had caused his death was not established. The clothing was eventually found under a nearby railway arch, and his bicycle 150 yards away, near Edgware Underground Station.

The accused man, when arrested in Ireland, had traces of the child's blood on his clothing. He subsequently admitted abducting the child and indecent assault, but denied manslaughter. At his trial he was nevertheless found guilty of manslaughter, abduction and indecent assault, and was committed to be detained at a psychiatric hospital without limit of time.

Chapter Eighteen

Child Murders

Murders of children are among the most distressing that police and pathologist encounter. The random nature of the crime makes it difficult for the miscreant to be brought to justice, although occasionally DNA identification may be unexpectedly successful.

To encounter two child murders separated by only three months is exceptional. Both were committed on a gypsy site by the same assailant. As is so often the case, the first murder occurred within a very short time of the child's disappearance – in this instance a 10-year-old boy, the crime somehow particularly tragic as he had been staying with his grandparents for the school holidays. He had been very keen to do so and overjoyed when his parents, who lived some distance away, had agreed. After spending three happy days playing in the grandparents' garden, he had ventured with his football the next day after tea on to a piece of waste ground a short distance from the house. His granny followed to join him some ten minutes later, but he was nowhere to be seen. About a quarter of an hour later she encountered two police officers, who were responding to reports by gypsies that they had found the boy's body on some ground adjacent to their site. A man was subsequently questioned by police, but he was alibied by a friend for that afternoon.

There was no doubt that the boy had been subjected to extreme force. His lips and eyelids were bruised and swollen and there was a large graze on the left side of the face and temple, caused, I thought, by his head being battered against the ground. There were lacerations across the back of his head, the skull was extensively fractured, and the brain had been fatally damaged. It appeared he had been hit by a brick or a piece of concrete. There were also signs of strangulation – a ligature mark on his neck had been caused by a piece of green tape. There were no signs of sexual interference.

Three months later I was called to examine the body of a five-year-old girl found in a gypsy caravan, some twenty miles away from the first murder. There were again signs of asphyxia, with a remarkably distinctive pressure indentation on the front of the neck in the form of a pattern of crossed swords on the skin; there were also grazes on the front and sides of the neck. The girl had, in gypsy tradition, been wearing several articles of jewellery, and in particular a pendant around her neck in the form of a trefoil or clover leaf motif, enclosed within a metal circle which was attached to a piece of cord. She must have been grabbed from behind by the necklace, which was then pulled firmly against the front of her neck to create the imprint I had found.

There was a bruise on the left wrist, probably as her arm was seized and twisted, marks on the front of the body due to pressure against the metal mattress in the caravan, and haemorrhage into the lungs, undoubtedly caused by severe pressure on the ribcage, which was bruised – a very unusual injury. There was also evidence of gross sexual assault, with bruising and tearing of the genitalia. She had been strangled, her chest had been traumatized, and she had been raped.

The man who occupied the caravan was traced to East Anglia and charged with her murder. On being further questioned about the previous murder, that of the boy, he admitted it, saying he had lost his temper with the lad – who he alleged had called him a 'gippo'. At his trial he was found guilty on both charges and given two life sentences. The judge, Mr Justice Miskin, recommended he should serve at least twenty-five years in prison.

When the man's guilt became apparent, the gypsy community of the area was outraged, and vowed to get even with him, saying he would die for the attacks. An attempt was made to ram a police car in which the accused was travelling to a police station, so these threats were taken seriously and his trial was switched from the provinces to London. One is fearful for his fate when he is eventually released into the community. Detective Superintendent Harry Clements, in charge of the case and an old friend of mine, told me after the trial that the murderer was a very dangerous sadist with a very low IQ, and that he had previous convictions for theft, burglary and indecent exposure.

An entirely different set of circumstances surrounded the death of a 10-year-old Ghanaian boy at the hands of his parents. The murder charge that followed led to a very unsatisfactory and highly unusual outcome – and only after two trials had taken place and a third was in prospect.

The boy was found in his bedroom at home, lying across his bed. He had been manually strangled by a right-handed grip; there was the imprint of a thumb on the right side of his neck, and other marks on the left side and back of the neck had been caused by the fingers. According to my criteria, he had died some time in the early hours of the morning, when both parents were in the home. The police were called to the house by the mother, who said there had been a burglary and the intruder must have been disturbed and killed her son. On questioning she changed her mind, alleging that her husband was responsible for the boy's death.

At the subsequent trial the husband was convicted of his son's death and sentenced to life imprisonment. A month later his wife received a letter from him beseeching her to tell the truth about the matter. After visiting him in prison she went to the police and said that she was responsible for the boy's death. The first conviction was therefore quashed. However, at the second trial, this time of the wife, she said that her confession was a false one, invented to help her husband.

After some nine hours' deliberation the jury failed to reach a verdict. This meant a third trial, because the original proceedings were now considered unsafe and untrustworthy. It is a strange feeling when one has to give the same evidence in a case in court twice, as one obviously cannot use exactly the same words and phrases as in the previous trial.

There was no third trial, as at its commencement counsel for the Crown, prosecuting the case, said that, after he had consulted the Director of Public Prosecutions, responsible for the management of trials, it was decided, owing to the confused circumstances and the tangled web of evidence previously heard, that no further evidence would be offered to the court. It was impossible to differentiate between the husband and wife in this matter.

A similar situation sometimes exists in the case of a battered baby when only one parent is charged. If there is sufficient evidence to do so, it is always more satisfactory to charge both parties. In this instance, of course, the father, found guilty at the first trial, was now acquitted and discharged; at the second trial the jury had been unable to reach a verdict. It was a strange case.

Chapter Nineteen

Nilsen: The Serial Killer

On Wednesday 9 February 1983 I was in the cutting-up room, as it is called, in the histology section of my department at Charing Cross Hospital Medical School, looking at some fixed tissues from a case. (I hasten to add that the term 'cutting-up room' is not slang for a place where bodies are dismembered or dissected, as in the anatomy department, but refers to an area where small pieces of tissue taken from current cases are examined and put aside for processing and later microscopic examination.) It was mid-morning – not unusual for me to be in the department on a Wednesday morning, as Wednesday was a day I was not required on the north London circuit and so could catch up on the administration of the department and the myriad of problems that could accumulate during the previous week.

'Mr Jay to see you, Prof,' said the departmental secretary. 'Mr Jay' happened to be Detective Chief Inspector Peter Jay, an experienced officer with a quiet sense of humour. He had brought me several strips of skin to examine. They were pallid, somewhat thickened, and indurated. They appeared to have been partially boiled or exposed to a tissue fixative, the skin having fatty tissue on the deeper surface and a few fine hairs on the upper surface. There were also four small bones to be examined. The superintendent of the mortuary to which these tissues had originally been taken had said they were from a chicken but this was not the case.

'It's human skin, all right,' I said. 'The fine hairs suggest the skin came from the neck area, and the bones are from a hand – two main bones and two fingerbones.' So advised, Jay returned to north London to await the arrival home from work of a Mr Nilsen.

The discovery of the bones was the culmination of a series of events that had disturbed a house in Cranley Gardens, Muswell Hill, north London, a conventional suburb for commuters with rows of neatly built three-storey Victorian houses. The view of the whole area from adjacent Alexandra Park, high up on the hill, gives the impression of a solid, large, well planned Victorian suburb. In the house in Cranley Gardens, the top floor was occupied by Dennis Nilsen, and the ground-floor flat was subdivided into two separate sections, in one of which lived two girls and in the other lived a girl and her boyfriend. The middle floor was empty. In recent years the house had to some extent deteriorated.

The previous Saturday, 5 February, an unpleasant smell had been noticed by tenants. They had notified Dyno-Rod, the well established drain-cleaning firm. The Dyno-Rod representative found a mass of fleshy material in the main drain. He consulted head office and, on account of the weather conditions – it was bitterly cold and dark – they agreed to leave matters to the following day. When he returned in the morning he found to his surprise that the drain was virtually empty. During the night the occupants of the ground-floor flats had noticed some curious doings – footsteps on the stairway and in the garden, and sounds of a drain cover being removed.

The disturbance was, of course, Dennis Nilsen making a last-ditch effort to clear away the evidence found in the drains. He said later – he had an acute and distinctive sense of humour –

that he had intended to clear the drain and replace its contents with Kentucky Fried Chicken. Meanwhile he had penned a letter to the landlord pointing out the deficiencies at the address – in particular that, when he flushed the toilet, those in the lower flats overflowed, indicating that the drains were blocked, with concomitant unpleasant odours. A well written letter.

His activities during the night had not been entirely successful. A mass of flesh that had previously blocked the drain was later found in a solid frozen mass in the wilderness of the rear garden. Meantime, Dyno-Rod submitted their account to the landlord. It itemized reaming and descaling the toilets, cleaning down to the manhole, and removing a large quantity of paper waste with a vast quantity of meat. As a rider, nicely put, a note was made of the broken and dangerous manhole cover. The bill came to £68.00.

Detective Chief Inspector Jay interviewed Nilsen as he arrived home that evening, asking him to account for the finding of human remains in the drainage system. Nilsen replied, 'Since when have the police been interested in drains?' Jay pointed out that the remains could only have come from Nilsen's flat, and also asked where any further human remains could be found. Nilsen, in his sitting room – a small attic room – pointed to the locked brown wardrobe and handed Jay the key. Under caution, he accompanied Jay to the police station. He would well have understood this procedure, having at one time himself been a probationary constable in the Kilburn area of north London.

During the drive to the station Jay asked Nilsen how many bodies they would be considering. 'Oh, fifteen or sixteen,' said Nilsen, causing the driver to almost lose control of the wheel. A nasty accident was narrowly avoided.

That same evening I made an initial examination of the flat and was struck by its fetid atmosphere – this although Nilsen always kept the windows open, even during the day when at work, partly for the benefit of his little dog Blip, who did not like being cooped up. (Blip, incidentally, was taken away and eventually died, although many people volunteered to look after him.) There may, of course, have been other reasons for this arrangement.

The case of Dennis Nilsen stands four-square with such earlier murder cases as those of Crippen, Ruxton, Haigh, Heath and Christie. It has a special niche in murder archives as it involved, so far as was known at that time, the criminal disposal of the largest number of persons by one man in British history.

I was fortunate – if one can use the word in this context – to be able to examine Nilsen's latest victim within a week of the man's death, as well as two other bodies which were later identified in the flat in Muswell Hill which he had been unable to dispose of satisfactorily following their dismemberment. It soon became apparent that it would be impossible to find the cause of death in two of the three cases, and that identification would also be a problem. Indeed, it was only in the case of Nilsen's last victim that the cause of death was ever scientifically established.

There was explosive interest from all sections of the press; such interest came close to contempt of court on occasions, and even at the end of Nilsen's trial a newspaper anticipated matters by reporting that the jury had come to a verdict some hours before they actually did so.

Dennis George Nilsen, aged 37, occupied the ground-floor flat in 195 Melrose Avenue, Cricklewood, north London, in 1976–81 and while there disposed of twelve men. Somewhat involuntarily – the house was being sold – he moved to 23 Cranley Gardens, Muswell Hill, some eight miles to the east, and there he strangled three more young men. In addition, over the same period of time, he made some seven unsuccessful homicide attempts on men who had been invited, for various reasons, to spend an evening with him or to stay temporarily at his flat. A total of twenty-two homicides or attempted homicides over the course of seven years leads one to an average of one victim every ten weeks; in actuality, of course, the time intervals between the crimes varied. All the men were either strangled or garrotted, usually following a session of heavy drinking of Bacardi and coke by Nilsen while he listened to rock music through earphones.

His work with the Manpower Services Commission often brought him in contact with the less well off and unemployed male section of society, and it was from this social grouping that he chose most of his victims – although not all followed this stereotype. One of those killed at the first address, in Melrose Avenue, Cricklewood, was a Canadian student who had intended to leave the country and unfortunately met Nilsen the night before his departure. At the time, his disappearance had been a matter of considerable interest and there had been a big investigation; however, his death was not confirmed until a thumbprint on a London Road Atlas found at Muswell Hill revealed his identity.

There may have been in Nilsen's mind a desire to rid society of certain persons but, probably more important, he appears to have been a lonely man who, bizarre as it may seem, kept his victims in his flat for as long as possible; in other words, he may have found them companionable – hence the title of the book on the case by Brian Masters, *Killing for Company*.

Nilsen's life began in Fraserburgh, Scotland, in November 1945. He was the second son of an exiled Norwegian soldier and a Scottish mother. The marriage broke up, and the mother subsequently remarried. She remained in contact with Dennis, who was regarded by her with considerable affection. In 1961 he joined the Army on a twelve-year contract and he was posted in 1964 to the Royal Regiment of Fusiliers in Germany, in the

Army Catering Corps, having obtained a City and Guilds catering diploma – perhaps this training gave him some knowledge of anatomy and skills in the dismemberment of a body. He was promoted to Lance-Corporal in 1965 in the Pioneer Corps and travelled widely – to the Persian Gulf, to Cyprus, to Berlin and eventually to Scotland, close to Balmoral, his unit on one occasion being involved in providing catering facilities to Her Majesty the Queen. Discharged in 1972, having served his contract satisfactorily, he was given a good-service record.

That same year he joined the Metropolitan Police and, after initial training, was posted to Q Division in northwest London, which involved the area of Cricklewood, including Melrose Avenue, where his first crimes took place. He found police work unsatisfactory, although logistically it gave him a good knowledge of this bedsit area of London and also a smattering of legal knowledge.

He left the police in 1973 and joined first the Department of the Environment and then, in May 1974, the Manpower Services Commission, where he was still working at the time of his arrest. His post had prospects and he became a minor official in his trade union.

Before considering the crimes in detail we should realize a significant difference between his Cricklewood home and the one in Muswell Hill. The former had a garden to which he had sole access; the latter was a top floor or attic flat. The house did have a garden, but he was virtually precluded from using it as a repository for human remains.

His Cranley Gardens flat consisted of a small kitchen with bathroom beyond, a bedroom and a sitting room. As noted, I went there on the evening of 9 February with CID officers who showed me their findings. A large wardrobe in the sitting room contained two plastic refuse bags. The first – a heavier bag – enclosed a large black bag, two white bags and a Sainsburys store container bag. Later at the mortuary I found that between them the two white bags contained the entire tissues of both sides of a human chest, cleanly dissected from the ribcage in an expert manner, while the black bag held a human torso from the neck to the lumbar region. The Sainsburys bag contained some internal organs. The second large refuse bag contained six smaller ones that between them held the upper half of a torso with the muscular tissues partially dissected away; there were arms but no hands. None of the victims found except the latest had hands or feet, which Nilsen removed.) There was also a decomposed skull devoid of tissue and a freshly decapitated head – Nilsen's last victim – with distinctive asphyxial type haemorrhages on the facial skin. Later a large plastic container bag in the bathroom, concealed under a wooden shelf, was found to contain a freshly dissected torso.

In the corner of the sitting room there was a large tea chest, inside which were some clothes and newspapers, a large white plastic bag and a large black plastic bag. The former contained a torso with some muscle tissue of the left leg partially dissected and most of the muscles of the right leg missing. The black bag contained a second bag and two blue ones, between them holding a skull with five neck vertebrae present, two upper arm bones, lower arm bones, and a pelvis or hip girdle, all more or less devoid of tissues.

A difficult task lay ahead. There were the major parts of two bodies plus a recently dismembered one, the latter being easily identified by fingerprints. According to Nilsen, the other two victims had died in March and September 1982 respectively.

A tour de force by Anne Davies of the Forensic Science Laboratory, Scotland Yard, Lambeth, led to identification of one of these men by matching blood-group substances still present in the muscle tissues with some original hospital blood-grouping work done of a man who, Nilsen said, had stayed in the flat.

The other body was also identified, again through a fine piece of detective work. A search was made on police and other files for people who had been missing since September 1982. A Mr Allen's disappearance was confirmed by his girlfriend, who said that before his disappearance he had fractured his jaw in a fracas when the police had had to be called to arrest him. He was taken to Charing Cross Hospital for treatment, where his fracture was stabilised with wire. Subsequently Allen removed the wires that had been inserted in his jaw, so the fracture had not healed in the normal way. On close examination of the jaw at post-mortem, the remaining fracture line was clearly evident, which became valuable evidence with regard to identification. Allen had also visited his dentist for an upper denture which he had never collected. With the collaboration of Mr Bernard Sims, forensic odontologist, we found that the uncollected dentures fitted the skull. Moreover, dental records and the original X-rays from Charing Cross Hospital provided further evidence of identification.

Cricklewood presented a much more difficult problem. The garden of the house was by now staked out and provided with the usual police protection. The soil in the area was sifted to a considerable depth, and the skeletal remains found were carefully collected into plastic bags. The adjoining wasteland, between the houses and the railway line, was also examined for bones. Eventually the entire collection was removed to Charing Cross Hospital for detailed examination and assessment. It was a matter of cleansing and sorting animal from human remains, with an effort being made to identify individual bones anatomically.

Nilsen's method of disposal of his victims was unusual. He left the body until rigor mortis had passed off, dismembered it and distributed the parts under the floorboards; as space there was limited he later removed the material progressively to the garden to make room for newcomers. He sometimes buried the body parts under surface soil, but later he started enormous bonfires which he topped with tyres, to disguise the unpleasant smell of burning flesh. After the fires had died down he used a roller to crush the remaining bones. In fact, the only unburnt bones found in the Cricklewood garden and surrounds were two sets of ankle bones, one complete in a victim's sock, and a few small complete bones; there were no long bones. The remainder were charred fragments, amounting to upwards of 2,000.

We knew the bones were all of young men, and Dr Jean Ross, Senior Lecturer in Anatomy, made it possible to identify certain bones, carrying out a detailed comparison of anatomical bones with bone fragments. After many weeks' work she was able to say there were ten identifiable fragments of bone from the upper limb, six being from the lower end on the left side, so at least from the anatomical identification we know there were not fewer than six bodies represented.

More out of interest than anything else, I tried out a method used by archaeologists to identify collections of bones found in ancient burial sites. Bones exposed to ultraviolet light fluoresce, and varying colours can be seen according to the different elements in the bone structure and on the surfaces. It is therefore possible to match bones from different places of origin to particular burial sites. We soaked bone fragments in a fluorescing pigment solution and then exposed them to a source of ultraviolet light. This proved unsuccessful for further identification, although an interesting academic exercise.

Neither was Nilsen's lawyer successful in his defence plea of diminished responsibility. The jury found Nilsen guilty on the six charges to which he had confessed. He was not charged with the death of Mr Allen, his penultimate victim at Cranley Gardens, although the other two victims were included.

Almost all the evidence presented at Nilsen's subsequent trial was based on the accused's own statements, so the entire investigation, legal and medical, was, curiously enough, the other way round from usual: we had to confirm Nilsen's statements, not disprove them, to substantiate charges of homicide. Any discrepancy between Nilsen's statements and the medical and forensic findings would immediately throw doubt on the veracity of the whole case, particularly as it is not unknown for a person to confess to crimes that he or she did not commit.

Had Nilsen chosen to remain silent – and he might well have done so but for careful police handling of his initial interviews – the deaths for which he was responsible, particularly those at the earlier address, might have gone completely undetected. Some idea of his activities and of his black humour are revealed when he mentioned to Detective Superintendent Geoffrey Chambers, in charge of the case, that, had he continued undetected, he would have reduced the population of north London by the year 2000 to the point that it would have been the subject of statistical comment.

There is a postscript. A year later I received a bone-like object from the attic of the house in Cricklewood. It had been found by plumbers investigating a leaking water tank. The press headlines the next day announced: 'NILSEN CASE REOPENED IN VIEW OF NEW DISCOVERY AT CRICKLEWOOD.' In fact, although the object resembled quite closely a bone from the arm, the Natural History Museum at Kew Gardens identified it as a variety of South American seaweed, found, curiously enough, on the Scottish seashore in the region of Aberdeen and around the Shetland Islands. It was an extraordinary quirk of coincidence that it had found its way accidentally into Dennis Nilsen's attic.

Chapter Twenty

Sexual Mishaps

Sexual activity should not be associated with a health warning, but in persons with a poor cardiovascular system there may be occasions when it can precipitate a cardiac arrest. American pathologists have coined the phrase 'death in the saddle' – a phrase that is seldom used in this country, and certainly *never* in a coroner's court!

Leaving aside the genre of sudden collapse during normal sexual activity, some deaths are associated with abnormal or unusual practices. They are well recognized by the public in general and the media in particular, and an investigation in the coroner's court is conducted with the utmost tact and speed. The hearing usually takes place before the appointed time for the court to sit, so that local journalists, if not national ones, seldom have the chance to garner a newsworthy account of matters.

The usual story is that of a young or middle-aged man found asphyxiated, with some form of restraint around his neck, his aim having been to cause himself partial anoxia and presumably heighten sexual pleasure. The scheme comes to a sad end when the restraint, usually a rope or cord, slips and tightens unexpectedly. Although such subjects are usually partially or totally undressed, they may be in female clothing; even so, they are generally heterosexual, not homosexual. The manner of their death is usually devastating to the family, who probably knew nothing about these proclivities. Such incidents in females are exceedingly rare.

A typical case concerned a 43-year-old man who, the evening of his death, had remained late in his office, ostensibly to work. He was found by his secretary when she arrived the next morning. It was a very unpleasant surprise. The body of her boss hung from a flight of stairs by a rope secured to a beam in the loft. Pornographic photographs lay on the floor, along with a small bottle which had contained chloroform, presumably to aid anoxia. On his face was a rubber mask, with apertures for eyes and mouth, giving him a rather startling appearance – even more so since this mask was white and resembled a rabbit's head. An apron-like suit of black plastic material on the front of his body was attached to a girdle of plastic around his pelvis, enclosing his penis. The autopsy showed the customary signs of asphyxia, death having been due to the rope slipping and compressing his neck.

At the inquest, witnesses spoke of the complete normality of his behaviour, his happy marriage and his successful business career. The coroner returned a verdict of accidental death.

Subsequently I received a number of letters from solicitors concerned about insurance policies held in his name, in particular clauses pertaining to fatal accidents. As the circumstances of his death were unusual, the various companies were adhering strictly to the terms of the policies and their definitions of a 'fatal accident', so the family's claims for a very substantial sum of insurance money were being resisted.

Reading through the letters and my replies explaining the case, I can only guess that I was being exceedingly naive in not demanding a fee for my assistance. Needless to say, no offer was made to me, and nor did they mention that they were prepared to pay for my opinion.

The companies holding the policies relied on a clause that the beneficiary of their estate should not benefit from any act which could not in normal circumstances be regarded as accidental. Moreover, he should have apprised them of his indulgence in such activities in the same manner as someone who participated in motor-racing, flying, etc., would inform the insurance company so that the premium could be adjusted. The companies therefore required an expert opinion as to how this accident had occurred and, in particular, whether I could tell from examination of the rope and associated equipment if he had habitually engaged in these activities or if this had been a one-off event. This interpretation of the policies relating to his death was interesting, and eventually the case went to a Court of Arbitration, where a satisfactory settlement was made.

Years ago, when the sexual nature of these incidents was not fully understood – before much was known about the use of partial anoxia to give a sexual rush – such deaths were regarded as suicides. Sir Bernard Spilsbury was the first pathologist to draw attention to the true nature of the condition. These accidents also occur with or without any sexual connotations in younger adults and teenagers who play or experiment with ligatures and ropes, not realizing the activities may be dangerous.

Other sexual mishaps are more complicated, and may involve the well known legal concept of *Volenti non fiat injura*, which in simple terms means that a person cannot claim on any loss or injury suffered if they give express or implied consent to a particular activity taking place. There is an apocryphal story of an uneducated country lad being called to the witness box in a case involving such matters. The judge addressed him: 'I expect you are aware of the meaning of this term?' The lad replied in broad country brogue: 'Of course, My Lord. Where I come from we speak of nothing else.'

An example occurred in a case examined by my colleague Dr R. Sarvesvaran. A 40-year-old man answered a notice placed in a shop window by a lady who advertised her availability, in particular relating to matters of 'restraint'. The implications were obvious, and the man duly attended her flat. Fortunately for her, as it proved, he brought with him an unusual shopping list of procedures which he wished her to follow to satisfy his sexual needs. They were twelve in number and, broadly speaking, were sado-masochistic – they included jabbing his body with high-heeled shoes and the use of a whip, a gag and restraint by a rope. There was an interval or half-time built into the schedule – the list specifically read: 'Leave me while you have coffee.'

When the woman returned to complete his requests she found him collapsed. The ensuing inquest returned a verdict of accidental death. She was lucky that he had provided written evidence of the circumstances surrounding his death.

A most unusual scenario involved a lesbian eternal triangle. At very short notice, I had to attend court to give an opinion on a head injury which had crippled one of a trio of lesbians, a deputy headmistress. The head injury, allegedly caused by her partner, a games mistress, had been sustained in the living room of a house in north London in August 1985. Both parties had worked at the same school.

The incident was initiated when, in the absence of the games mistress, a third woman spent the weekend helping the deputy renovate a house which she had inherited. The guest precipitated a sexual liaison. The games mistress became aware of this when she returned to the household the following week. That morning the guest left the house to get a newspaper. When she got home she found the deputy headmistress lying in a pool of blood. During her absence, a space of some ten minutes, the deputy had been attacked with a claw hammer.

The games mistress, alone in the house with the victim, maintained that, after taking a bath, she heard a groaning sound downstairs and found her partner lying on her back with a hammer by her side. The deputy headmistress was in a coma for six days in hospital, after which she was left brain-damaged, paralysed and confined to a wheelchair.

The games mistress was subsequently accused of causing and inflicting grievous bodily harm. The trial took place, most unusually, in the Royal Courts of Justice in the Strand, the Central Criminal Court being closed for August. Because of the venue, there was an unaccustomed informal atmosphere for a criminal trial. My recollection is that the incident was initially regarded as the result of a fall from a ladder while decorating, and that it was only subsequently, as the tangled web of the relationships surfaced, that investigators began to suspect it was something more sinister.

I was asked for my opinion as to the manner in which the deputy headmistress had sustained the blows, and in particular about the pattern of bloodstaining on the uncarpeted floor and the wall – matters usually dealt with by a forensic scientist. The police had previously investigated whether the deputy head-mistress could have suffered a head injury following the fall from the ladder, and also the theory that an intruder could have been responsible.

My view was that the blood splashes on the floor and wall were consistent with the hammer having been wielded by the accused. As the assailant drew the hammer overhead and delivered it downwards in a blow against the deputy's head, it had produced a pattern of bloodstains in the shape and form of exclamation marks on the wall.

The accused was found guilty and sentenced to seven years' imprisonment, the minimum sentence the judge could impose, balancing the grievousness of the crime with her previous good character. She had recently lost her father, and the relationship which had developed between her lover and the third woman

had kindled jealousy so overwhelming that she had uncontrol-
lably attacked the deputy, all but destroying her life.

A remarkable group of serial murders with a sexual background
occurred in southwest London during the spring and summer of
1986. Between April and July of that year seven elderly people
who lived on their own in the area were found killed in their
bedrooms, all the murders being committed by one man. The
ages of the victims varied from 78 to 94; three were women,
four were men. One possible other victim lived in north London,
and one 73-year-old man attacked in June had fought back and
escaped his attacker's clutches – so there were up to nine
victims in total. In each case the victim's bedclothes were in a
normal position, pulled up to the level of the neck. There were
no obvious signs of a struggle or of a forced entry from the
street. In fact, the first victim was thought to have died naturally
until it was noticed that a television set was missing; at that
point the death became the subject of a CID investigation, and
its true nature became evident.

All the deaths were due to manual strangulation, with some
evidence of pressure across the mouth. In five of the cases – two
men and three women – there was evidence of sexual interference and assault (that is, buggery).

It was a particularly worrying time for the CID. On 29 July
1986, an hour after midnight on a warm evening, I went to a
quiet road just off Fulham Road, near Putney Bridge in west
London, not far from the Roehampton Club. The small flat of
the victim, Florence Tisdall, was on the ground floor, and it was
believed that the killer had gained access to it via a window left
open so her aged cats could go to and fro. The victim was 80
years old and unable to walk without a Zimmer frame, found in
another room. As with previous victims, she lay in bed wearing
a nightdress. A blanket, now across her legs, had been found
covering the body up to face level. There was a pillow beneath

her bed, and other bedding and clothing on the floor nearby. There was no sign of a struggle.

Death had occurred some twelve hours previously. At examination I could see grazes and bruises on her neck, in keeping with pressure from fingers. More important, there was a fracture of the cartilage of the voicebox on the left side, with bruising of the deep tissues of the neck on the right side, all consistent with manual strangulation. Bruising of the lips and mouth was suggestive of pressure, causing suffocation, and there were extensive asphyxial haemorrhages in the eyelids. There was no direct evidence of sexual interference. The usual collection of specimens for the laboratory was documented, signed and sealed in plastic bags.

The previous victims had lived south of the River Thames in sheltered accommodation, and it had fallen to my friend and colleague Hugh Johnson, who worked in that area, to make the examinations.

The eighth victim, the man who escaped with his life after the intruder panicked and fled, was able to give evidence of the attack and to pick out the assailant at an identity parade. Further, thumbprints of the assailant had been found in the houses of two victims, at the scenes of two of the other deaths, and in the survivor's house.

At the Central Criminal Court it was stressed that, aside from the direct evidence that was present in only three of the murders, there had been close if not identical findings in all the others. If the accused was found guilty of one murder, it was the Crown's submission that the striking similarity of the remaining cases would enable the jury to return a verdict of guilty involving all victims. There was no evidence of robbery; it was a matter of the wanton murder of all seven people.

The accused, 24-year-old Kenneth Erskine, of no fixed abode, was found guilty and sentenced to Broadmoor mental institution. He was a lonely drifter, longing for fame, living in a fantasy world, with perverted desires to kill elderly people. An odd feature in a couple of the cases, including that of Mrs Tisdall, was that a picture frame had been placed face-downwards on the chest of drawers.

Chapter Twenty-One

Forensic Puzzles

It is not as uncommon as one might suppose for it to be impossible to ascertain a precise cause of death. An autopsy may not reveal it, and at the inquest the coroner's verdict must therefore be 'unascertained'. The word 'unascertained' should not be confused with 'unascertainable', which latter might suggest that either the pathologist or the coroner had the omniscience of the Almighty. Perhaps, on second thoughts, there are one or two medical men who would fit into this category . . .

A typical example would be the sudden collapse of someone of considerable age, living alone, who was unable to go out except for a little shopping. In the deaths of young people, investigation may be hampered by the inability of the pathologist to carry out toxicological analysis – which might be particularly significant in a young person – or analysis for alcohol, as the latter is useless when the body has decomposed. My impression is that deaths whose causes are decreed to be unascertained are increasing in number, perhaps as pathologists are becoming less dogmatic about ascribing them to vague or unproven diagnoses.

Occasionally unascertained causes of death are associated with a tinge of mystery.

During early July in the very hot summer of 1976 I went to a solidly built Victorian house in north London, preceded there by the coroner's officer. Always smartly dressed and with a jolly rubicund face, well groomed white hair and a briefcase, this man was sometimes mistaken for the coroner or pathologist as he went on his investigations. He had a rich sense of humour and, anticipating the situation that I would encounter in the house, did not tarry at the scene. The scene of death was an attic loft on the third storey of the house. As I clambered up, I noticed a skylight window overlooking a small but pleasant garden with two deck-chairs. A powerful pair of binoculars lay on the skylight windowsill.

In the darkened recess at the far end of the attic I could just make out a prone body, the face lying against the joists. The house owner, 91 at the time, had not been seen for four days, and had been reported missing. A search of the house had proved fruitless. His body had been found by accident in the loft eleven days later.

The approach to the area where he lay was separated by a wooden door from the larger area of the loft, the entrance obscured by a couple of bed heads, a chair and an old trunk, so access to the body was quite awkward. The area had been investigated after a young female student who occupied a room below had noticed some discoloration on her ceiling and, on closer inspection, a small peephole through it. This peephole coincided with the position of the deceased's head on the other side. With the binoculars on the windowsill at the entrance to the attic, it suggested that the old gentleman was a peeping tom who had habitually watched sunbathers in the gardens of the neighbouring houses during that long, hot summer and, more particularly, had spied on the young student in various stages of undress in the room below.

It was only with some difficulty that I crawled into the area to view the body, and it was even more difficult for others who followed me to remove the corpse, covered as it was with unimaginable numbers of maggots and flies. The old man was in a resting position, face-down towards the peephole, wearing a vest; his trousers and underpants had been pulled down to his thighs. Perhaps the excitement had proved too much for his ageing heart. We never knew as there was precious little tissue left for examination. There was no sign of injury.

Another attic death the following year, 1977, was even more mysterious, although again no criminal activity was involved. The deceased was an easy-going man, 37 years of age, who left home on 13 January to travel to work. Although he arrived there as usual, he was seen leaving shortly afterwards – but never alive again. For eight months his disappearance was a complete mystery. A cursory examination of his house had been made by police at the time to try to find any documents that might lead them to his whereabouts. His body was discovered by chance by his wife's brother-in-law, who had gone to place some boxes in the loft. It was hidden behind a water tank and was in a completely mummified condition, the loft environment being dry and warm. The reason for his death remained as mysterious as his disappearance. There was nothing in his life to account for his behaviour.

Once again I clambered into a loft. He was lying on one side of the water tank, fully clothed, with a briefcase, containing sandwiches and correspondence, in his hand. A plastic bag over his head had been secured under his chin by a piece of cord. It was clear he had gained access to the loft by a stepladder, which he had drawn up after him.

I made as full an examination as possible, bearing in mind that the only finding relevant to his death was the plastic bag. Plastic-bag asphyxia is unique in that there are no associated asphyxial haemorrhages, as the plastic covering occludes the air passages very rapidly.

At the subsequent inquest, after considering the possibility of

an open verdict, the coroner decided that, owing to the circumstances of his death and the plastic bag, the man had taken his
own life. But we will never know for sure.

At the other end of the scale was the body of a man of 35–40
years of age found in 1978 at the bottom of a ventilation shaft
in Terminal 1 at London Heathrow Airport. It was in August, a
busy holiday period. This was a curious place in which to find a
body. The concourse had been roped off following the discovery of a damp patch on the floor next to the sloping cover of
a ventilation shaft. The man must have, in some way, descended
from the top via a long, permanent steel inspection ladder.

The geography of the area where he was found was complicated. The body was wedged at the lower end of the shaft,
between its metal cover and the panelling that separated the
shaft from the passenger terminal. How long he had been there
was unknown, but probably it was a week or two. He was
dressed in a short brown overcoat, checked shirt, pants but no
trousers, and a shoe and a sock on one foot. His hands were
clasped together in a resting position. Post-mortem changes had
developed, with some discoloration and loss of skin surface but
no evident injuries. Further examination was unhelpful, there
being no signs of asphyxia, natural disease, foul play or any
other condition that could have caused his death. I came to the
conclusion that he might have succumbed to lack of oxygen or
water.

Identity was easily established – he had a passport. He had
arrived from Canada some three weeks beforehand, extended
his stay at a Hyde Park hotel, and left there on the last day of
July. His suitcase had been deposited at the airport the following day.

I had previously viewed the shaft from the top, some fifty feet
from the ground – fortunately I didn't have to clamber down.
The airport authority discovered that the area had been occupied

by airport workers as a makeshift dormitory, unknown to the authorities, so it was certainly possible for someone to have gained access to it. But how had he reached his final resting-place? Not only was the cause of his death unascertained, but the circumstances surrounding it were unknown. An unfathomable and absorbing case, but with no evidence of foul play.

It is part and parcel of a pathologist's caseload to give an opinion on a wide variety of forensic cases and problems, almost always involving a court attendance. Not so in a case that came my way in November 1988 when I received a letter from a man convicted of grave criminal assault and rape, in prison pending his appeal. He had written to me on the advice of a police surgeon and asked me to give my opinion on the massive volume of court documents and evidence relating to his case.

He had been accused of committing, in July 1987, a serious offence on a 5-year-old girl whilst on holiday in Jersey, Channel Islands. It was a strange, sinister and complicated story.

The accused had been out drinking, and returned to his hotel room, where he allegedly fell asleep. On waking, he went down-stairs to watch television, having followed the girl's uncle into the room where the television was. Shortly afterwards the little girl ran into the room and pointed to the accused, shouting that he had strangled her. According to a statement she made later, the man had put his hands around her neck and placed a pillow on her face. When she was examined by the police surgeon, he found numerous small haemorrhages in the skin of the face, indicative of asphyxia and in keeping with an attempted suffo-cation. She also said, on being questioned, that the man had touched her between the legs.

The police surgeon's examination revealed bleeding in that area, with a scratch evident around the vaginal entrance. In court it was discussed whether the injury to the vaginal area was due to a finger, a penis or a tampon, and on balance it was thought to have been caused by a penis, although no semen was found on the swabs taken from the victim. The deputy bailiff summed up for the jury, dealing with every aspect of the case, and asked them to consider a charge of 'grave and criminal assault' if the pillow was used as described by the victim and also if there was evidence of rape or indecent assault. At the trial in April 1988 the jury brought a unanimous verdict of guilty on both charges, criminal assault and rape. In January 1989, at the appeal hearing, the accused was acquitted of rape but the conviction for grave criminal assault was left standing.

I thought the damage to the genital area could have been caused by a finger or foreign body, and as noted there were no seminal stains found, so perhaps the appeal court verdict had taken account of my opinion. Apart from the girl's statement, the sole evidence of the accused having been in the little girl's room was that his shorts had been found there.

It is highly unusual for a forensic pathologist involved in a case to be approached by a prisoner, although in fact I have had one other similar occurrence. This time it came as a result of the accused having received, quite correctly, three letters I had written to the law firm which had represented him, outlining my views. He wished to contact certain experts to whom I had referred in one of the letters, and also asked if the petechial haemorrhages on the child's face could have been the result of hysteria. Far from that being so, the child was lucky to have survived. Death could easily have occurred, and the prisoner's sentence would have been for murder.

It was fortunate that a most puzzling case I was called to on a bitterly cold morning in December 1965 was resolved using the technology of the time. A decade later, the investigation of the man's death would have had the advantage of more modern forensic techniques. Albert Willerton was a night watchman in a factory west of London which produced and stored cables.

One night in December 1965 he failed to report to his control point, and a search ended when his body was found in a large storeroom. He lay on his back, heavily clothed, his head partly concealed and wedged in a corner between stacks of drums. His hands were tied together across the front of his body, and his ankles were also secured by string. A break-in had been reported in the early hours, and a check revealed that a quantity of tin ingots and copper rods had been stolen.

Apart from some superficial pressure marks on the wrists and ankles, the only injury was a two-inch cut with abraded edges – a laceration – extending half an inch into the tissues behind the right ear but with surprisingly little evidence of haemorrhage in the adjacent area. Subsequent examination showed a considerable degree of thickening of the coronary arteries of the heart, as well as the scar of a previous heart attack in the muscle. There was no sign of asphyxia, strangulation or suffocation, or any evidence of a struggle. From external appearances he could have collapsed from a heart attack while confronting intruders.

Having excluded a skull fracture, I was surprised to find a large, recent haemorrhage at the base of the brain – clearly the cause of death. However, it was impossible to exclude a natural cause for the haemorrhage; quite often haemorrhage is the result of a rupture of a small developmental aneurysm (a weakness in the wall of the vessel) rather than trauma.

At that time pathologists knew little of the exact mechanisms of such an injury but, following observation and research by colleagues here and in the USA, it was realized that a blow to that area of the neck, below and behind the ear, could cause sudden death. Vertebral bodies of the spine high up in the neck contain a small canal within which is a thin-walled artery that supplies blood to the base of the brain. A sudden jar or blow to the overlying tissues may result in a tear in the vessel wall and a massive haemorrhage. This phenomenon may occur through ill luck and under the most unlikely circumstances, such as a transient superficial contact – as seen in a cricketer I examined, who seemed just to sway backwards to avoid a short pitched bouncing ball and then collapsed, from all appearances due to a heart attack. Examination showed a classical haemorrhage, no doubt caused by minor contact with the ball as it sped by, brushing against the skin of his neck.

Nowadays a routine procedure in a suspected case would involve radiology of the neck, following injection of a radio-opaque substance to visualize any leak of blood into the tissues or a breach of the vessel wall. Subsequently the tissues would be dissected and examined for a fracture. But of course we could not do that then.

In due course four men were arrested and charged with causing the man's death and with theft of material from the factory. They were sent for trial to an assize court. At the trial the judge, Mr Justice James, said it was unfortunate they had been committed on a charge of murder without any evidence to justify it, accepting Prosecution Counsel's view that there was no intention to kill and the death was unintentional. The accused men pleaded guilty to stealing the ingots and wire.

Whether the deceased had sustained a blow on the side of the neck or had slumped or collapsed against the sharp edge of a metal ingot will never be known.

There were similarities, not as to the cause of death but in terms of the demise, in another case some twenty-two years later. Albert Smith, the same age as Albert Willerton, was found in roughly similar circumstances, lying on the floor of a back room in his terraced house in north London, fully dressed and also, on initial examination, without evidence of serious injury. He had not been seen for several days, being discovered when police entered the house.

When I arrived at the scene, dusk was falling on a fine September day. The deceased was lying between an old armchair and a table, the only free space available in the small room, almost wedged in position, his coat pulled up to the line of his shoulders, as if he had been dragged into the room from the hallway and his left arm had caught against a table leg. There were two ties around his neck and a third on the floor nearby. One tie, a patterned grey one, lay quite loosely around his neck with a simple fold-over knot. The second, a nylon tie, had a very tight small knot and lay firmly against his neck, although loosely enough that a finger could be interposed between it and the skin. There was no evidence of a struggle or asphyxia. Discoloration of the skin of the neck had occurred due to developing post-mortem changes, with a faint impression of a mark on the skin, virtually encircling the neck. There was no sign of drugs or alcohol, or of exposure to carbon monoxide, and no sign of any significant natural disease.

As in the case of the first Albert, there was not a great deal to show for my investigation, but the results were not consistent with a natural death, partly due to the posture of the body (unlike a natural collapse) and partly due to the unexplained ties around the neck. I formed the view that it seemed likely he collapsed as a result of some form of pressure on his neck – vagal inhibition.

My evidence was explored over two sessions of the magistrates' court following the arrest of a young man in connection with causing Albert Smith's death. An astute senior QC had been engaged on the young man's behalf, and I anticipated a lengthy cross-examination. As we have seen, vagal inhibition is a rare but well recognized event, resulting from transient compression of the neck; in simple terms, it results from the reflex stimulation of a nerve from the brain which controls heart rate. It is usually associated with an element of surprise, sometimes fright or even terror.

The defence hinted that it might have been possible for the deceased to have tried to strangle himself, a view with which I could not agree. Usually self-inflicted manual compression of the neck, even with a tie, and without other means of constriction, does not cause death, as the victim becomes faint or dizzy and loses his grip.

The most significant witness in the case was a man who said he knew the accused and three days before the body was found had met him in the local pub. It had been near closing time when he had spoken to the accused, and he'd noticed he'd gained a Mohican-style haircut. The witness had asked the young man where he had acquired it, and been told he had done it himself while drunk. The accused had then asked the witness to lend him some money, apparently for drink, but the witness had refused. The accused had next said that he wouldn't be around for much longer anyway, as he had killed someone the previous night – which remark the witness did not take seriously at the time. Some three weeks later, however, he reported the conversation to the police. Perhaps he had seen a notice of the investigation of the death of Albert Smith in the newspaper.

The accused was committed for trial at the Central Criminal Court, but was there found not guilty due to lack of evidence connecting him with the man's death.

Stabbing is the most common form of homicide in this country, varying from one strike unfortunate enough to pierce a vital vessel or organ, usually the heart, to multiple stab wounds where some fifty injuries may require documentation; in one instance where a double-edged knife had been used (a bread knife) there were over a hundred such injuries. A stab wound whose depth is longer than the external width implies a sharp instrument, usually a knife, which the police will find either at the scene or after a prolonged search, or not at all. Accidental stab wounds do occur, but these are usually associated with an occupational hazard – the butcher's knife that slips. That leaves a small number of suicidal stab wounds which become self-evident due to the circumstances and the exclusion of an outside assailant. Occasionally, however, there may be difficulty in distinguishing suicidal stab wounds from homicidal ones.

The body of a 35-year-old student found in his flat near Shepherds Bush Green, west London, was kneeling against the seat of an armchair. A friend had called to see him, said he saw the body, touched it and it immediately fell backwards. It had been fortuitously and delicately balanced in a state of rigor mortis. There was a knife on the dressing table on the other side of the room, some ten to twelve feet away, and a large pool of blood around the armchair.

The puzzle was that the deceased was on the other side of the room from where the knife was found. To those attending the scene this circumstance indicated the death could be homicide. There were four stab wounds in the region of the heart on the left side of the chest, each an inch across, very close to each other; they had caused a fatal internal haemorrhage. Reconstruction showed that the student would indeed have been able to stab himself while looking in the dressing-table mirror next to where the knife was found, then to stagger and collapse across the room on to the chair. Finally, contraction of his muscles into a state of rigor maintained his position until his friend arrived – all in all, an unusual sequence of events.

Information was received that he had suffered from depression and two days earlier he had informed the Samaritans of his intention to take his own life.

An additional feature was that his chest was bare of clothing, the shirt open; the hallmark of a suicidal stab wound is almost invariably exposure of the chest in this manner.

The latter principle was vital in a case in 1967. It was an unusually tragic one. At 7 a.m. one day I was called to a detached house in the suburb of Barnet, north London, with Detective Chief Inspector Colin Saxby, an amusing and enthusiastic officer whom I had met on many occasions.

A 53-year-old woman lay on her back in the downstairs cloakroom. She was wearing a bloodstained nightdress, and a German war dagger was just outside the cloakroom door. Spectacles and dentures were in place, and from temperature measurements it appeared that she had died the previous evening. Her husband had been taken to a local hospital with neck wounds that required surgical attention and treatment, and the CID was naturally anxious for him to make a statement, particularly as it seemed likely that he had stabbed his wife and then his own neck. An arrest appeared imminent.

There was an extensive distribution of bloodstains in various parts of the house. The principal areas involved were on the back of the front door extending downwards from the lock to the ground, on the telephone by the door, and on the staircase wall and banister; the trail continued on the landing carpet, around the landing light switch and on the left-hand side of the double bed in the main bedroom, also on the carpet between the front of the bed and the adjacent wardrobe. Many blood spots were present on the upturned dressing-table stool, which had small fine cuts on its surface. There was heavy bloodstaining of the bedclothes.

The deceased had superficial bruises on both arms and a cut in the web of the left index finger, but the fatal injury was to the front of the left breast, where two incised wounds were seen, respectively an inch and a half and two inches long, the main one being a stab wound which had penetrated the chest to a depth of seven inches, entering the main artery that runs from the heart to the lung. The wounds were hidden by the top margin of her nightdress which, on examination, was not involved or pierced, indicating that it had been pulled down before the wounds had been inflicted, an unlikely scenario for a homicidal attack by her husband.

In the interviews of her husband, who recovered in hospital, a remarkable story unfolded. There had been domestic friction for some time and a further argument on the night of his wife's death. It had been partially resolved before the husband settled down to sleep. He awoke, so he maintained, to find his wife standing over him wielding the SS dagger subsequently found downstairs. He realized that he had been stabbed a number of times in the neck while asleep. Jumping out of bed, he attempted to wrest the dagger from her, failed to do so, but picked up the dressing-table stool to use as a shield against further attacks. He then staggered downstairs. His wife had preceded him, going to the cloakroom where she was later found. Failing to make a 999 call on the phone – understandable, considering his plight – he opened the front door and reached the house next door, where the occupant, a doctor, gave him first aid before calling an ambulance.

Blood-grouping confirmed that all the bloodstains except those in the cloakroom were from the husband, confirming his story, so his wife had sustained an unusual but characteristic self-inflicted wound – in fact, she had committed suicide following her attempted murder of her husband and the case was not one, as originally thought, of a husband murdering his wife.

I believe I got the truth of it. Everything depended on the nightdress being intact and free of tears from stab wounds.

When is a murder hunt unsuccessful? Obviously when no arrest is made in connection with the crime, but just occasionally when the medical findings are ambivalent. Such was the case in the death of an ageing man in north London in the late 1960s. The event was strange, and capable of various interpretations. The CID regarded it as a murder mystery. I was unconvinced of the medical findings in the matter.

John White, an 86-year-old man, was found slumped in his chair in the front room of his flat. He was fully dressed, with a dressing gown over his clothes. Although his face was pale and free of all asphyxial or suffocative changes, there was a gag around his mouth, knotted at the back of his neck. His wrists and ankles were tied together in a strange way, as the same length of material ran from his bound hands to his bound feet – he was trussed up, one might say. His wrists had been secured by double knots and the gag was a folded white scarf, secured tightly by a granny knot across his mouth. His spectacles lay on his lap, and he had his deaf aid around his neck.

He was a slimly built man with quite marked arthritic changes. No bruises were evident. Curiously enough, as is often the case in such circumstances for a man of his age, his heart was not as enlarged as one might have expected, but the lungs were very moist, in keeping with heart failure. In the absence of any injury indicative of an assault, all one could say was that he had developed acute heart failure which had been precipitated by shock, associated with being gagged and tied up.

Uncle Jim, as he was known, was a friendly old chap, according to neighbours. It was said that he had come into some money and that, in the few days before his death, there had been something worrying him which he would not divulge. The neighbour who found him said the television was on, the man was in the chair as described, and the place was, as he put it, ransacked – drawers and small boxes had been turned over. The television sound was blaring – perhaps to stifle Uncle Jim's shouts?

That was as far as the case went. There was nothing to show any money had been stolen, although initially it looked as if that was the case. Uncle Jim's death completed a trilogy of men found dead in highly suspicious circumstances, but in this latter case there was no evidence of burglary. It was even suggested to me that the trussing up was part of some form of sado-masochistic exercise.

The findings were heard at the local coroner's court, where a verdict of unlawful killing was returned.

The unravelling of forensic puzzles is part of their fascination, but I was unprepared for the events when, late one August evening in 1981, I was called to a flat in north London. CID officers were already there. The flat belonged to one John Dean, a Native American by birth. An ex-girlfriend of his had gone to the flat, been unable to get in and informed the police. What the police discovered was truly bizarre.

The flat was well furnished and had several rooms, but it was the bathroom that was the focus of our interest. Lying in the bath in a few inches of water was the naked body of a woman, her head and shoulders resting against the back of the bath, well out of the water. Some signs of decomposition were developing across her shoulders. There was a curious dark indented oval mark in the middle of her forehead and, beneath it, as I found later, an airgun slug or pellet with a lot of bruising spreading around the side of the head to the back. The skull was not damaged, but the impact of the pellet could have stunned her. There were further unpleasant surprises awaiting my examination: a distinctive irregular indented brownish area of damaged or abraded skin around the left nipple, probably a bite mark, and also damage to the anus, which was torn, with some of the skin bruised. The anal damage was the result of either buggery or the forceful use of some instrument. She had not been strangled.

The bathroom floor was littered with various objects connected with her death. There were two champagne glasses, one broken; two bottles of Charles Hiedsieck champagne; a telephone set, the handpiece lying separate and broken; a small portable convector heater; a large hacksaw; and bloodstained knickers. The lavatory pan contained a length of sanitary-towel-type material incorporating white elastoplast and cotton wool, which had obviously been used as some form of gag. Other clothes were in the adjacent lounge, where also a packet of airgun pellets lay on a chair and a half-empty bottle of vodka sat on a small table with a partly smoked cigar.

Three questions arose. In what order had these bizarre events

occurred? What was the cause of death? And who was responsible? Although she might have gone to the flat of her own
volition – as it transpired, she had been another girlfriend of the
man subsequently found responsible for her death, John Dean –
she had probably been kept there against her will, being
sexually assaulted and shot with an airgun. Finally, as we found
from examining a gas pipe in the bathroom cupboard that had
been sawn across, she had died from inhalation of natural gas,
as confirmed by laboratory tests.

In the corridor leading to the flat was the entrance to a large
storage area containing packing cases. There, suspended from a
metal rafter, was the body of John Dean, who had hanged
himself. It was a case of murder followed by suicide.

The secrets of the flat were revealed and the horrifying nature
of the girl's death was heard later in the coroner's court. The
court heard that John Dean worked for an import–export firm as
warehouse manager – hence his adjacent flat. He had had a
relationship with the girl, and had lived with her in north
London, but she had broken off the relationship the previous
year. Two months before their deaths he had once more met the
girl, Ann Belan, who was found in the bath, but in the final week
of their lives she had refused to see him. She must have gone
along to the flat voluntarily, but then been held there and met
her death. Dean had threatened to take his own life in the past.

Chapter Twenty-Two

The Mystery of Rudolf Hess

The mysterious death in prison in Germany in 1987 of Rudolf Hess has been, over the years, the subject of much speculation, most recently in the definitive biography by Peter Padfield and, from a medical point of view, by Hugh Thomas, a consultant surgeon posted to Berlin and in attendance on Hess when he remained the last inmate of Spandau Prison, identified only as Allied Prisoner No. 7. My involvement with this case was entirely due to Hugh Thomas, who wrote asking my opinion on the cause of death as related by two separate post-mortem reports, one on behalf of the Four Powers and the other on behalf of Hess's family.

To understand the questions hovering over Hess's death one must go back to the evening of 10 May 1941. Earlier that day a twin-engined ME110 fighter had taken off from Augsburg, an airfield close to the Messerschmitt works. The pilot, Rudolf Hess, aged 47, was Deputy Führer of the Third Reich, second only to Hitler in importance. During the First World War he had served initially in the infantry, transferring to the Air Force in the last year and becoming a fighter pilot. Maintaining his enthusiasm for flying afterwards, he won the Round the Zugspitz Mountain Air Race in 1934.

Unlike many of the Nazi hierarchy, Hess was well educated,

with a university background. He had first met Hitler in the 1920s, becoming embroiled, dazzled and mesmerized by the movement and the man, initially as Hitler's secretary and then rising to the pinnacle of German nationalism.

Hess's flight destination was the northwest coast of Scotland. Darkness had not completely fallen at 11 p.m. when a Messerschmitt roared across the sky south of Glasgow towards Dungavel, Dungavel House being the home of the Duke of Hamilton.

The pilot ejected by parachute, landing near the village of Eaglesham, and the aircraft crashed nearby. Hess's mission was an attempt to broker a peace deal between Britain and Germany, and for that purpose he wished to contact the Duke of Hamilton, also a distinguished aviator as well as a Member of Parliament who served in the Royal Air Force. Hess thought he had met him at the Berlin Olympic Games of 1936, when he had been known as the Marquis of Clydesdale, having not yet inherited the dukedom.

It is at this point that the plot thickens. In his provocative 1988 book *Hess – A Tale of Two Murders*, Hugh Thomas raised serious questions about the true identity of the pilot. As part of the evidence set out in that book, Thomas investigated the distance involved in Hess's flight from Augsburg to Scotland and the likelihood of his fighter plane having been able to reach its destination. He concluded that it was not Hess who had landed but his double. The markings on the fuselage of the plane leaving Augsburg appeared to differ from those seen on the crashed plane in Scotland, and this led to the belief that it was a second night fighter, based in Denmark, that had finished the apparent journey, with, of course, a different pilot – Hess's plane having been forced down or shot down en route.

Hess's seeming arrival in Britain led to a brief statement on the radio; no further official statement was issued. Reaction in Germany was entirely different. Hitler was incensed by his deputy's apparent defection, and a statement was issued saying that Hess was mentally deranged, had a progressive illness and had been forbidden to fly so must have crashed somewhere on an unauthorized flight. No official identification seems to have been made.

From Scotland the man was taken briefly to the Tower of London for interrogation; then to Mytchett Place, a Victorian building near Aldershot; and subsequently, in 1942, to Maindiff Court Hospital in South Wales. Later still, after the war's end, he was sent to Nuremberg to stand trial with other Nazi leaders.

He was a remarkably difficult, uncooperative prisoner. The several psychiatrists who saw him thought he could have a schizophrenic personality with paranoid tendencies and amnesia. At one time he attempted to harm himself by pinching the skin over his heart and stabbing it with a kitchen knife, producing a wound which required a couple of stitches.

At the war trials in Nuremberg, Hess, then 53 years old, made a statement in which he claimed responsibility for his past misdeeds and stated that he had previously feigned amnesia. He was found guilty of war crimes and, with six other prisoners, on 18 July 1947 arrived in Spandau Prison to spend the rest of his life there. He died at the age of 93.

From 1966 onwards he was the sole prisoner at the prison. It was at this time that he was examined by Hugh Thomas, then working as consultant surgeon at the RAMC hospital in Berlin. Thomas's subsequent reason for doubting that the prisoner was really Hess was the absence of certain scars which he had expected to see during an X-ray examination relating to a gastro-intestinal complaint. Hess had been wounded in the First World War on three occasions. In 1916 he was hit by shrapnel in the left arm; he sustained a second arm wound the following year. In August 1917 he was severely wounded, spending four months in a number of hospitals, being discharged in December. This last was a near-fatal rifle-bullet wound and, as Hess described it, it ran under his left shoulder and out through the back of his chest. It was likely that, following the injury, he would have required surgical exploration, an incision and drainage. According to his wife he often referred to the scar – his war wound – but he never mentioned it during his captivity. It is *possible* that the entrance and exit of the bullet might have been obliterated by the passage of time; that said, it is surprising how persistent scars are from wounds, let alone from operations.

In August 1987 the prisoner became extremely feeble. He could read very little as he had poor eyesight, and his left arm and hand were of little use – he could not move the arm above the horizontal plane. His right arm was little better, and it was only just possible for him to comb his hair. His sense of balance was grossly impaired.

On 17 August he went for his usual exercise into the prison garden at Spandau with an escort. After lunch and his usual afternoon nap, at 2.30 p.m. he was taken by the duty warden back into the garden and along the garden path, and an hour later the warden took him to a shed or summerhouse, where the man sat with Hess for a few minutes before being called to answer the telephone in the main cell block. There is no record of him asking for any writing materials while in the summerhouse; even so, examination of his clothing two days after his death revealed what purported to be a suicide note.

As for the shed itself, the roof sloped to a height of about eight feet and the eave over the door was some six feet from the ground. The shed was full of clutter, including several lengths of electric flex left by a workman.

When the warden returned he found Hess lying on the floor in a crumpled position, half-sitting, bent forwards, with his knees up to his chest, propped against a folding chair. The warden realized that Hess was dead, and saw a length of flex around his neck. Help was immediately summoned and resuscitative procedures were attempted.

A Special Investigation Branch team arrived, and concluded that Hess had managed to throttle himself by passing the ends of the flex through the roof structure, putting his head through the loop, and pulling hard down, so that his breathing was occluded. It was an extraordinary action for an aged man to carry out – one with a feeble grip and limited arm movement.

A brief statement was made to the effect that Rudolf Hess had taken his own life, although a further investigation to ascertain the cause of death would be carried out.

That investigation took the form of an autopsy performed by Professor James Cameron, who was civilian consultant to the Army in forensic pathology. He was assisted by an RAMC specialist pathologist; also present were a number of prison governors, representative of the Four Powers, and medical advisers, together with five Special Investigation Branch men who had been initially involved in the examination of the shed.

The body was formally identified by the hospital command-ing officer, and only the medical men and the SIB men remained for the autopsy. The body was still fully clothed. The previous day, when X-rays had been taken, permission to remove the clothing had been withheld. It is very unusual for a deceased's body to remain fully clothed while being X-rayed as such a procedure leads to poor quality and definition of radiographs. It was decided to record the autopsy on closed-circuit television, no photographs being taken – again a remark-ably unusual procedure to adopt in the circumstances.

Prior to the full autopsy, the clothing was of course removed, and it was now that the ostensible suicide note was found in the jacket pocket. There is little justification for accepting the note as genuine. Hess's son, Wolf Rudiger Hess, certainly did not believe that his father would have written such a note immediately before his death, and thought it might have been written many years earlier, when Hess had thought he was dying – it referred to matters occurring before his family had visited him in prison.

The external examination started with an investigation of the body under ultraviolet light. This has been used in the past to develop the image of bruises or injuries, particularly old ones. It is a procedure which some pathologists regard as unreliable and of uncertain value. Cameron found a number of external injuries: on the left side of the neck; on the back of both wrists; evidence of recent hospital therapy, probably injections; also marks of resuscitative measures on the front of the chest, particularly on the left side, associated with multiple rib fractures.

The significant injuries were an oval bruised abrasion over the top of the back of the head, with underlying deeper bruising. These marks were regarded as being due to a fall or an impact on the ground. An alternative explanation would be that they were due to a blow to the back of the head. On the left side of the neck a fine linear mark, three inches long, was visible, but no other measurement of its position in relation to other structures was made, and of course no photographs were taken.

Curiously enough, there was an old scar on the left side of the chest. Although its nature was unspecified, it was almost certainly due to the minor wound self-inflicted by Hess some years earlier using the kitchen knife.

Further internal examination showed bruising or haemorrhage into the strap muscles on the left side of the neck, with bruising over the left side of the angle of the jaw and inside the back of the throat. The report concluded that the latter was consistent with resuscitation attempts. There was excessive bruising of the right side of the voicebox in the area of the main (thyroid) cartilage; a fracture of the upper part of the wing of the cartilage was confirmed by radiology. There was further deep bruising behind the voicebox, over the right side of the neck.

Examination of the other internal organs revealed no significant findings.

The conclusion reached at the autopsy was that there was no

evidence of natural disease, there were marks of resuscitation, and that there was an asphyxial element in the cause of death, this being confirmed by the number of haemorrhages in the eyelids. The mark on the skin of the left side of the neck was in keeping with a ligature, and injury to the voicebox, with the fracture, indicated compression of the neck. The cause of death as given officially was asphyxia due to compression of the neck due to suspension.

The weakness of the report lies in the fact that there was no elaboration, elucidation or discussion of the meaning of the word 'suspension'.

Such was the concern of Hess's family that a second post-mortem was requested. This was carried out at the Medico-Legal Institute in Munich by professors Wolfgang Spann and Eisenmenger. This translated report was made available to me by Hugh Thomas, so I had both reports to study.

Spann described a reddish-brown mark running obliquely from behind the left ear, across the throat below the cartilage of the larynx, and to the right side of the neck, with a very signifi-cant double mark across the back of the neck, running almost horizontally. Spann was in general agreement with Cameron as to asphyxia and suspension, but he drew attention in particular to the mark across the back of the neck, which had not been mentioned in the original report. This mark cannot be explained by classical hanging, and cannot be produced by pressure across the back of the neck when the neck is placed on a support at autopsy; such a mark would be only transitory.

In the case of any mark on the neck, the distinction between hanging and strangulation is critical, and depends on the angle of compression by a piece of rope or flex. In hanging, the mark runs in a V-shaped form diagonally down the sides of the neck, across the front and up into the nape of the neck, where it disap-pears at the point of suspension on whichever side of the neck that takes place. In ligature strangulation, the mark runs horizontally, without a mark of suspension – and this appeared to be the case with Hess.

Spann's report was remarkably detailed, outlining the significance of the two different forms of asphyxia caused by pressure on the neck. He stated that his findings were more likely to indicate strangulation than hanging. In no circumstances could they be interpreted as the results of a typical hanging, although he could not exclude an atypical form of hanging, as sometimes occurs when the deceased lays his neck against a ligature, thereby passively compressing the neck – this is sometimes seen when the deceased has been suspended from a very low point.

The report leads me to the conclusion that, in his examination and conclusion, Spann made a pertinent and very significant contribution to the mystery surrounding the death of Rudolf Hess.

One month after the event, the Four Powers issued a statement that Rudolf Hess had hanged himself from a window latch in a small summerhouse in the prison garden using an electrical extension cord which had been kept in the summerhouse for use in connection with a reading lamp.

It is, of course, possible that atypical hanging had occurred, but if so an explanation is still required as to how it was carried out. The British Governor of Spandau, Tony Le Tissier, in his book *Farewell to Spandau*, indicated that the flex found on Hess's neck was knotted to the window handle of the summerhouse and Hess had only to loop the loose end around his neck, secure it with a slip knot and slide down the wall, differing from the previous statements of the SIB and the Four Powers. However, even this manoeuvre would require a degree of mobility and dexterity which Hess lacked. General enfeeblement, advanced age and arthritis combine to make it unlikely that he took his own life.

The flex and the garden shed, as well as Spandau, were later destroyed. There was no question that the pathologists carried out their task with circumspection, but perhaps the political background and significance of the occasion meant that the prisoner's death did not lend itself to a satisfactory post-mortem investigation.

Numerous books written on Rudolf Hess have concentrated on reasons for his flight, the possibility that it was not Rudolf Hess who landed in Scotland but an impostor, and the attitude of British authorities to his arrival and subsequent fate. Documents from the Public Record Office have also been released.

Much less consideration has been given to the thesis that Hess was murdered by order of the British government.

Whilst it may be seen as a far-fetched and an unlikely scenario, the views of his son and my own consideration of the two post-mortems with an analysis of the alleged method of suicidal hanging leave considerable doubts as to the truth of the matter.

Although suicidal hanging can occur from a lower point of suspension such as a chair, the resultant mark on the neck and internal tissues are few owing to the limited drop of the event; certainly nothing to compare with the bruising in the deeper neck tissues that was found at the post-mortem. So this is more puzzling. Hospital therapy mentioned in the initial autopsy report may have involved injections into the neck tissues, carried out almost two hours after Hess was found. It would have been most unlikely to cause significant haemorrhage, particularly into the deeper neck tissues. It is unusual for haemorrhage or bruising to occur during the process of hanging, even less so in atypical hanging when trauma to the tissues is minimal. It is, however, a feature of strangulation. Bruising to the top of the head is also unlikely to occur in hanging, unless there has been a substantial impact against the head during the deceased's fall. Doubts must remain on the reliability of the official statement given concerning the death of Rudolf Hess.

Bibliography

Board of Trade, *Civil Aircraft Accident: Report of Public Inquiry*, CAP 270, 27 October, 1963

Board of Trade, *Civil Aircraft Accident Report*, CAP 322, 3 July, 1968

Board of Trade, *Civil Aircraft Accident Report*, 14/76, 29 November, 1975

Camps, F.E., and Purchase, W.B., *Practical Forensic Medicine*, Hutchinson Medical Press, 1956

Coogan, Tim Pat, *The IRA*, Harper Collins, 2000

Cornwall, Rupert, *God's Banker: The Life and Death of Roberto Calvi*, Unwin Paperbacks, 1984

Cottrell, Richard, *Blood on their Hands: The Killing of Ann Chapman*, Grafton, 1987

du Rose, John, *Murder Was My Business*, W.H. Allen, 1981

Gillard, Michael, *Calvi: the tests that might point to murder*, the Observer, 31 January 1993

Goodman, Jonathan, ed., *Masterpieces of Murder*, Robinson, 1992

Goodman, Jonathan, & Waddell, Bill, *The Black Museum*, Harrap, 1987

Le Tissier, Tony, *Farewell to Spandau*, Ashford, Buchan & Enright, 1994

Masters, Brian, *Killing for Company: The Case of Dennis Nilsen*, Cape, 1985

Owen, Richard, *Mafia face charges over Calvi murder*, The Times, 24 July 2003

Padfield, Peter, *Hess: The Führer's Disciple*, Cassell, 2001

Picknett, L., Prince, C., Prior, S., Brydon, R., *Double Standards*, Little, Brown & Co., 2001

Popham, Peter, *God's Banker was throttled then strung up, inquiry finds,* Independent, 22 February 2003

Ransom, David, *The Blair Peach Case: Licence to Kill*, Friends of Blair Peach Committee, 1980

Simpson, Keith, *Forty Years of Murder*, Harrap, 1978

Thomas, Hugh, *Hess – A Tale of Two Murders*, Hodder & Stoughton, 1988

Willan, Philip, *New clue turns up in 'God's Banker's death,* The Guardian, 14 October 2002

Internet References

Question of the week – The First Calvi Mystery: Was his death suicide or murder?
www.edwardjayepstein.com/question_calvi.htm
New tests 'say Calvi was murdered' BBC News
www.news.bbc.co.uk/1/hi/world/europe/1936830.stm
Ban looms over Vatican bank movie BBC News
www.news.bbc.co.uk/1/hi/entertainment/film/1897387.stm
Report on Calvi autopsy returns spotlight to Vatican Bank scandal American Atheist
www.atheists.org/flash.line/vat13.htm
God's banker murdered in Mafia plot Bruce Johnston
www.telegraph.co.uk/news/main.jhtml?xml=/news/2002/10/26/wcalvi26.xml

Index